D1383261

TRAVIS
+
MACE

:)

A Mile at a Time

A father and son's inspiring Alzheimer's journey

of love, adventure, and hope

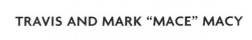

TRAVIS AND MARK "MACE" MACY

WITH PATRICK REGAN

imagine!

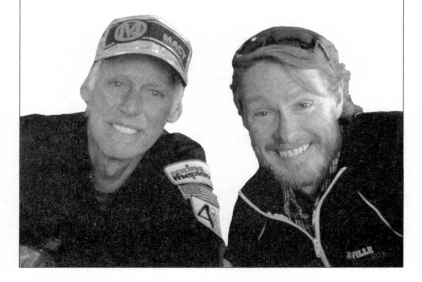

Copyright © 2023 by Mark Macy, Travis Macy, and Patrick Regan

All rights reserved, including the right of reproduction in whole or in part in any form. Charlesbridge and colophon are registered trademarks of Charlesbridge Publishing, Inc.

At the time of publication, all URLs printed in this book were accurate and active. Charlesbridge and the authors are not responsible for the content or accessibility of any website.

An Imagine Book
Published by Charlesbridge
9 Galen Street
Watertown, MA 02472
(617) 926-0329
www.imaginebooks.net

Library of Congress Cataloging-in-Publication Data

Names: Macy, Travis, author. | Macy, Mark, 1949– author. |
Regan, Patrick, author.
Title: A mile at a time: a father and son's inspiring Alzheimer's journey of
love, adventure, and hope / by Travis Macy and
Mark "Mace" Macy with Patrick Regan.
Description: Watertown: Charlesbridge Publishing, 2023. | Summary:
"A father and son participate in 'the World's Toughest Race,' the
Eco-Challenge Fiji, as the father battles Alzheimer's Disease."
—Provided by publisher.
Identifiers: LCCN 2022000874 (print) | LCCN 2022000875 (ebook) |
ISBN 9781623545550 (hardcover) | ISBN 9781632892492 (ebook)
Subjects: LCSH: Macy, Mark, 1949– | Macy, Travis. | Alzheimer's
Disease—Patients—Biography. | Fathers and sons—Family relationships. |
Endurance sports.
Classification: LCC RC523.2.M33 .A3 2023 (print) | LCC RC523.2.M33
(ebook) | DDC 616.8/3110092 [B]—dc23/eng/20220318
LC record available at https://lccn.loc.gov/2022000874
LC ebook record available at https://lccn.loc.gov/2022000875

The display type in this book is set in Agenda One
The text type in this book is set in LTC Caslon Pro
Printed by Maple Press in York, Pennsylvania
Production supervision by Jennifer Most Delaney
Jacket and interior design by Lilian Rosenstreich

Printed in the United States of America
(hc) 10 9 8 7 6 5 4 3 2 1

Dedicated to the Alzheimer's community

FRIEND: Your buddy is still the same person, just a little different.

SPOUSE: Dig deep—and remember you've got to take care of yourself to take care of your partner.

CHILD: May something here support your journey.

DIAGNOSEE: As Dad says, "Keep the faith and never give up."

Long may you run
Long may you run
Although these changes
Have come
With your chrome heart shining
In the sun
Long may you run

—NEIL YOUNG

FOREWORD

I FIRST ENCOUNTERED Mark "Mace" Macy in the Utah desert in 1995. I was producing the first-ever Eco-Challenge, a multidiscipline, multiday adventure race that had drawn athletes from across the globe. Along with those 250 competitors were twenty film crews; two helicopters; hundreds of crew members; reporters and camera crews from MTV, NBC, ABC; and a massive contingent of print media reporters and photographers. The scene on the sunbaked ground was exhilarating, intense, and borderline chaos.

In the midst of the madness, I met a lot of competitors. The vast majority of their faces have been lost to the mists of time. Mace, I remember. This was an alpha-type crowd. I knew the type well from my time as a British Army paratrooper: tough, bombastic, prone to a certain bravado. That wasn't Mace. He was quiet and amiable. Lean and tan, he certainly looked the part of an ultra-endurance athlete. But what really struck me about Mace was his eyes. There was steel in those blue eyes. They told a story. A short one. "I don't quit."

The story of that first Eco-Challenge is well recounted in the pages of this book, but the short version is that Mace started as a member of one team, and when half of that team succumbed to the grueling 370-mile gauntlet of climbing, running, biking, horseback-riding, and paddling, Mace and a teammate made a field decision to join up with survivors of another depleted team. Right there in the desert, the newly formed team of weary but still willing warriors chose a perfectly apt name: the Stray Dogs. Together, they finished the race, and over the ensuing years the team's members, including "Mace" Macy, would go on to become legends of the adventure racing world.

I got to know Mace and his teammates a little bit better every year. To be honest, they were never a serious podium threat. They were perennially up against younger, stronger, faster, flashier teams, but like hungry stray dogs, they kept showing up. To me, the team captured the true spirit of Eco-Challenge. When I conceived the race, I was never caught up in the winning and losing. The point was to tell stories—to capture the interpersonal dynamic within a group of committed people willing to sacrifice their individual well-being and comfort for the greater collective goals of a team.

And what a story the Stray Dogs were! If the old dogs weren't favored to win the race, they were always favorites of fans, the crew, and the locals wherever we went. Over the years, I became a fan not only of Mace's grit but his spirit and humor as well. Of course he suffered in those races—all the competitors did—but the tougher it got, the more Mace seemed to enjoy it. He truly was made for this stuff.

As the Stray Dogs continued to add chapters to their story, the Macy family was living out another, more personal, story. Mace's wife, Pam, would undergo three separate organ transplants over the course of twenty-seven years, all while she and her husband raised a family of biological and adopted kids, the eldest of whom, Travis, had followed in his father's footsteps to become a world-class athlete himself. Trust me, it's a story worth hearing from the source!

In 2019, twenty-four years after the inaugural Eco-Challenge and after a seventeen-year hiatus—during which, well, let's just say I stayed busy—we brought the Eco-Challenge back.

Leading up to that event, which was to be held in the jungles and mountains of the Fijian Islands, I recall reviewing a list of team applications. Some of the names I recognized, but most I didn't. It had been nearly two decades, after all. Still, I shouldn't have been surprised—scanning the list, there it was, that old familiar name: Macy. I can't recall if, at the time, I noticed there were actually two Macys on the list: Mark (old "Mace" himself) and Travis.

I would soon learn the remarkable course of events that led Mark and Travis, father and son, to Fiji. That story—so well chronicled in this book—has it all: pathos, adventure, humor, despair, and joy in equal measure.

Most of all, though, it has heart. Faced with Mark's shattering diagnosis of early-onset Alzheimer's less than a year before Eco-Challenge 2019, Mace, Travis, and Pam made a bold decision. Alzheimer's would not stop Mace from doing what he loved. They decided to stay in the race. Was it risky? Absolutely. Foolish? Quite possibly. But the fundamental question was this: Is there more risk in taking on a seemingly impossible challenge or in folding up the tent and going home, wondering forever what might have been?

The through-line of my own story has always been one of risk taking. To pull off that first Eco-Challenge, I had to bluff, cajole, beg, borrow, and put everything I had on the line. People—smart people—thought I was insane to go all-in as I did. In Mark Macy, I see a kindred spirit. His insistence on listening to his heart rather than the voices of the doubters has led him to places most people will never see.

In Mace's story—and that of his family—I have found an inspiring reminder that with love, determination, and teamwork, the most formidable challenges can be overcome. Living the life you love is always worth the risk.

—MARK BURNETT
Award-winning producer and creator of
Eco-Challenge, World's Toughest Race, Survivor, The Apprentice, The Voice, and *Shark Tank*

A NOTE TO THE READER

OUR STORY BEGINS with an entry from Mace's journal, which he started after receiving an Alzheimer's diagnosis. We have also begun each chapter with an excerpt from the journal, which is a personal, passionate expression of Dad's resilient spirit (not to mention his ongoing sense of humor in the face of dire circumstances). While Dad tried to write a few of the entries by hand, he dictated most of the content to Mom because deterioration of fine motor skills rendered handwriting and typing impossible.

Thanks for reading and being part of our team. And if you're also going through something tough, please know that we're part of your team and we share this story with hopes that it helps you.

—*TRAVIS*

MY NAME IS MARK MACY. *I am fifty-six years old and today I was diagnosed with Alzheimer's disease.*

My doctor, a neurologist, told me to get my affairs in order, since ALZ is invariably fatal. He advised me to not spend time worrying about this diagnosis, to instead take vacations, maybe go on a cruise with my wife, Pammy.

I told him: THIS IS BULLSHIT.

My wife just told me I am sixty-four, not fifty-six. Maybe it's not complete bullshit.

Five months ago I donated a kidney to a stranger. You have to be in perfect health to be an organ donor. I am one of the fittest people around; I run and bike and swim most days and certainly am as fit and healthy as any fifty-six-year-old. (My wife just told me again I'm not fifty-six years old. I am not making this up, that really just happened.)

I finished day one of my Alzheimer's diagnosis with a significant decision: I didn't cause this disease, I'm not embarrassed to be one of the millions of people suffering from it, I'm not going to hide from it, and I'm going to share our story with anyone who wants to listen. Pammy, my son Travis, my daughters Katelyn and Dona, and I will dedicate ourselves to fighting this horrible disease that kills people all over the world.

I'm going to share our story with anyone who wants to listen and share in our excitement when I beat this thing.

—Mark Macy's journal
October 16, 2018

INTRODUCTION

FORTY-TWO HOURS AFTER starting most races, you've long since crossed the finish line, showered, slept, had a nice dinner, and returned home. Forty-two hours after starting the World's Toughest Race: Eco-Challenge Fiji 2019, we were just getting going on an epic, human-powered, 671-kilometer journey. Our team of four experienced endurance athletes—Dad, Nellie, Shane, and I—had paddled from dawn until dusk on day one, using map and compass to navigate a traditional Fijian outrigger sailing canoe—the *camakau*—from Fiji's main island in the western Pacific to a smaller island where we trekked for hours up and over a jungly mountain range.

The next morning, we paddled the heavy boat for another five grueling hours into a headwind. The small island we targeted resembled the stereotypical "tropical island paradise" of movies and survival jokes: ringed by beaches, crystal waters, and coral reefs—all of which would have been exciting to see provided we could ever get there. "I swear," Dad exclaimed as he paddled hard, despite growing pain in his sixty-five-year-old back, "that fucking island is getting farther and farther away from us!" The rest of us couldn't really tell if the island was actually floating away from us or if Dad's perception was distorted by his Alzheimer's disease.

Hours later, with the wind finally in our favor as we headed back toward mainland Fiji full of the bula spirit, we hoisted the sail and cruised over the ocean at a snappy pace. With Shane steering from the stern and Nellie tending the sail, Dad and I rested, taking in some needed calories (saltwater-soaked trail mix and energy bars... tasty!). Feeling present in the moment as I often do in intense outdoor situations and very happy to be there with my father, I turned in my seat at the bow to see Dad behind me. He was smiling and looking off in the distance, clearly feeling comfortable and at ease in this journey, widely recognized as one of the most challenging endurance events on earth. Alzheimer's was making things in daily life increasingly hard, and we knew the rest of the Fijian racecourse held a dizzying range of perils and tests. But for this moment Dad and I were at peace as our eyes briefly connected and we shared a smile.

Looking deeply into my father's bright blue eyes, I thought, "I'll make sure we get through this okay, Dad." Transitioning to new familial roles can be tough. I know it was for me, particularly when Alzheimer's hit my dad—not only a father but also a friend and adventure companion and rock and motivator and grandfather—at a relatively young age. But I felt strong and up to the task, proud to hear myself think, "I'm ready to take care of you out here, Dad."

SLAM!

Less than a second later, I was upside down in the ocean, disoriented and flailing my arms. I gasped for breath but gulped saltwater instead. A brief panic ensued until a hand—strong, sure, steady—grasped the back of my life jacket and yanked me to the surface.

"Hey, Bud! You OK?"

The voice was Dad's, and so, of course, was the hand. Our boat had capsized due to a rogue wind gust, but Shane righted it while Nellie swam around grabbing our packs. The old guy with Alzheimer's may need some help tying his shoes or organizing his race gear, but here in the thick of it he remained strong and steady, instinctively reaching out to grab his child before thinking about anything else.

Twenty-nine years earlier. I am seven years old, walking away from my family's house in Evergreen, Colorado. With each step, the light from the house is swallowed more deeply by the dark. Real, starless mountain dark. I don't like the dark and what it can hide—bears, mountain lions, ghosts, The Unknown. I reach out my hand instinctively, and it is instantly wrapped in the strong, warm grasp I know so well. The opposite of The Unknown. Security. Strength. Love. Dad.

This, I now know, is where it began. Where it ends, well, we are bound to find that out, together. Our journey has taken us to places washed in sunlight and draped in darkness. The Fijian archipelago and its surrounding waters serve as an unusual backdrop for our Alzheimer's story, but I'll just admit this up front: Dad and I are pretty unusual guys. At least that's what a lot of people think.

In the fall of 2020, amidst a global pandemic generating uncertainty for all, millions of people around the world watched part of our story—a very small part—play out over ten episodes on Amazon Prime. Yes, the World's Toughest Race was a made-for-television event, but it was also very real—full of real dangers; real drama; and, like us, real people. For Dad, it was almost certainly the end to an amazing run. He is one of the few people to have participated in eight of the original Eco-Challenges, beginning with its inception in 1995 and running through 2002, the last year the race was held before a seventeen-year hiatus during which its creator, Mark Burnett, concentrated on developing other reality programming, most notably the cultural phenomenon *Survivor.*

Dad was a stalwart competitor in those races, as he has been in a staggering number of other ultrarunning and endurance races over his adult life. He has challenged himself physically, mentally, and emotionally, at levels few people have experienced—or, frankly, could even comprehend. His resilience, strength, and spirit inspired me at an early age to follow in his footsteps and become a professional endurance athlete. Dad has always shown me the way.

But something changed a few months before we were invited to participate in the reincarnated Eco-Challenge. In October 2018 we got the news: At sixty-four, Dad had been diagnosed with early-onset Alzheimer's disease.

Alzheimer's. No prevention, no treatment, no cure. That was the conventional wisdom. But Dad, as you will learn in this book, is not a conventional person. He decided—and we decided as a family—to fight this fight with everything we had. He decided to live fully instead of throwing in the towel.

By the end of our Eco-Challenge adventure, viewers worldwide got a little glimpse of the heart, strength, humor, and resilience of the man I've always looked up to (and still do). But the story of our Alzheimer's journey goes far beyond what the cameras captured in Fiji. From that first dark day of Dad's diagnosis right up to today, Dad, Mom, and I, along with the rest of my family, friends, and "teammates," have chosen our own approach to dealing with this insidious disease. Our approach will certainly not be appropriate for every victim of Alzheimer's, but our story, I believe, holds universal truths. And my greatest hope is that our story will help bring light, hope, and understanding to families who have faced the same thing we have. Alzheimer's is very much The Unknown. Finding that steady hand reaching out to you in the darkness can make all the difference.

SOUTH PACIFIC OCEAN, FALL *2019*

ONE

I have done many hard things in my life. Now's the time I've been training for. I've gotta step it up and do whatever it takes to save my life. And I will.

—MACE'S JOURNAL

THE TWENTY-INCH WHEELS of my little kid's mountain bike kept grinding over the rough mountain road, the faint but steady sound of skittering pebbles regularly punctuated by my dad's fortifying words: "Keep hammerin', Bud! You can do it!"

We had the road—which meandered up the foothills right outside our house—to ourselves. I gritted my teeth, stood on my pedals, and kept my eyes focused straight ahead. Despite the beauty of the surrounding woods, my eyes were locked on the knobby back tire in front of mine, and the powerful calves that drove it forward. I was five years old, and I wasn't about to quit hammering. I was following my dad up a mountain. It may have been the first time, or perhaps it is an amalgam of memories, but either way, it would be followed by countless more ascents over the decades. Dad and me. Hammering away.

To know me, you've got to know my dad. Ever since my earliest memories, my dad has occupied a space all his own. Sure he's changed and aged, like all of us, but my image of my dad today isn't that far from the image I had of him when I was following him up that road at five years old. Tall, lean, strong, tanned—that's the physical. Funny, nurturing, relentlessly positive, tenacious—that's the emotional. For all he's changed in my thirty-plus years of really knowing him, he may as well be carved out of granite. He's that solid, that consistent.

But he wasn't always my dad, of course. He forged that rock-solid personality during his own childhood, growing up in Livonia, Michigan, a suburb of Detroit that lies just west of the city.

> I grew up in a typical suburban neighborhood of four-bedroom brick houses with short-cut green grass lining all the streets. All the kids rode their bikes on the sidewalks and streets. We rode our bikes to school, carrying our baseball gloves wherever we went. I had an older brother, Greg, who I idolized. He was four years older than me and told me it was his obligation to teach me manners. This meant pushing me around and only letting me play baseball with him and his friends if there weren't enough people.... Greg was a successful attorney but unfortunately died of alcoholism at age fifty-six. My sister, Michelle, three years younger than I (then and now known as Boo), pretty much tagged along behind me as I tagged along behind Greg.
>
> I always wanted to be like my dad, and still do. My dad was a perfect father. He was a classic guy of the fifties; he had joined the army at an early age to fight in Europe. Remarkably enough he fought in the Battle of the Bulge, and like many men of

his generation, never mentioned it to any of us.
It finally came out when he was in his eighties.
Most important to me, my dad was always around
to play catch, throw a football, coach my teams...
and he attended the hundreds of sporting events of
mine over the years, including sitting in a cold car
all night long waiting for me to finish the Leadville
Trail 100.

I guess wanting to be like your dad runs in my family.

Unfortunately, alcoholism runs in my family too. Both my dad's mom and his brother died of the disease while in their fifties. Losing his mom when he was so young and living with her alcoholism while he was in school were the dark clouds over what Dad describes as an otherwise sunny childhood.

My aunt Boo (Michelle) likewise recalls a mostly idyllic suburban upbringing. The Macy home was one of the first to be built in a new subdivision, and nearby woods and a creek provided endless opportunity for adventurous outdoor play. She looked up to both her brothers, but in Mark (my dad) she had her first best friend and protector.

I was very fortunate to have Mark as a brother.
I was always a tomboy, and he let me tag along
with him whatever he did. He always watched out
for me. If anyone picked on me, he would defend
me. I remember a time when the bully of the
neighborhood said something mean to me. Mark
picked up a rock, turned around, and whipped it
at him... and then he got in trouble. But I knew he
was always there for me.

We didn't have kids over to our house because

we never knew if Mom was going to be drinking...
we'd always meet friends on the corner or at their
houses. At times Mom tried to go to AA meetings,
and she'd sober up for a while but then start
drinking again. It was just this endless pattern. She
was in and out of hospital... but back then people
were quiet about that sort of thing. And Dad never
talked about it.

My mom was a very strong woman—I truly
believe that. She was just living in an age where
the woman stayed home and raised the kids. She
gave up her job in retail merchandising—she could
have been a very successful woman, but she gave
up everything to have kids and stay home with
kids, and I think she just lost herself, you know?
After ten or fifteen years of raising a family, she
didn't feel like she could go back and start over
again. A lot of women felt that way... and I think
she had a hard time with my dad and his lack
of emotion. That was probably a big part of the
frustration too. My mom's dad was an alcoholic.
My dad's mom was an alcoholic, so it's obviously
ingrained in the family. I think Mom just fell into
that and lost herself. Mom was pretty athletic
too. She's the one who taught us all to play ball...
I remember playing catch with her in the yard.
She'd always go to all our sporting events... which
wasn't great sometimes, because she'd be drunk up
in the stands, yelling.

But Dad was definitely a role model for all of
us kids. He was hardworking and respected by
his colleagues, but he was quiet and didn't boast
about what he did. I think Mark just saw an inner

strength in him and a "don't quit" attitude, along with the intensity of pushing yourself to the limits. Push, push, push, and don't stop. That "don't quit" stuff... he ingrained that into us. You start something, you do your best at it and finish it. Dad was the root of the family and held us all together.

In addition to their parents, Dad, Aunt Boo, and Uncle Greg had another adult in the house: Bump Bump. Anna Marie Weisenberger was their maternal grandmother, who came to live with them late in her life because she needed support. The details are hazy, but they recall a "very old" woman (she was actually in her fifties and sixties) who stayed mostly upstairs and dished out loads of love for her grandkids (she called them all "kid") in between talking with characters on the black-and-white TV. Dad remembers her saying the moon landing couldn't possibly be real and regularly asking him to "please tell those people over there" (who didn't really exist) to leave the room. Things were much different back then, but if she were alive now I think Bump Bump probably would have been diagnosed with Alzheimer's or something similar. Thankfully, Dad and Boo remember her as loving and happy until the end.

Even if his brother, Greg, didn't always let him play ball with the big kids, Dad became a standout athlete just the same. He participated in nearly all the school sports—baseball, basketball, football, soccer—but, surprisingly, he says that he always hated running and wasn't very good at it. "I always thought running was for people without any athletic ability," I remember Dad saying. "It's what the coach makes you do when he's pissed off at you."

Athletics came easily for Dad, as evidenced by the way he walked onto his college's lacrosse team just a few days after learning the game existed. He tells the story of walking across the campus at Michigan State and seeing some guys with sticks throwing a ball back and forth.

"I asked one of the guys, 'What are you doing?' He said, 'We're playing lacrosse.' And I said, 'Can I play?' He said, 'Do you know how?'"

The answer was no, of course, but Dad waited till practice was over and approached the coach about joining the squad. A few days later he was playing in his first game. It was also the first lacrosse game he had ever seen.

Dad swears that his own dad never missed a game out of the hundreds he played in his school years, even traveling to MSU's away games. I'd find that hard to believe had my own dad not maintained a similar perfect record of attending my games as a student athlete. And, frankly, I can't imagine missing one of my kids' games either, should they turn out to be athletes.

It's probably fortunate that my grandpa was at Dad's games, because an alarming number of them involved an injury. Over the course of his early athletic career, Dad sustained multiple concussions and contusions. The first one he recalls involved an errant swing at a tossed baseball. His friend missed the ball but hit him square in the forehead. Out cold. Head protection was inferior even in contact sports in the 1960s and '70s. Dad recalls that the lacrosse helmets they used in college felt like they were made of cardboard.

I got hurt real bad playing lacrosse once. I got hit right in the forehead with a ball early on in a game. My parents had arrived at the game a little late, and they pulled up at about the same time as an ambulance. My parents asked who the ambulance was for and found out that I had been knocked unconscious. To show you what an easygoing guy my dad was, I remember when they got to the hospital, my dad looked at me and said, "Merrick [his nickname for me], you okay?" I said, "Yeah," and he said, "Well, okay, we'll see you then." That was it. I ended up spending a couple days in the hospital, but he didn't get real excited or scared.

Another unfortunate but memorable head injury happened during one of Dad's Little League baseball practices. My grandpa coached a lot of my dad's teams, and one of his frequent cocoaches was a player for the Detroit Redwings hockey team. Dad and the boys on the teams called him Mr. G. "He was a good guy," recalls Dad, "but he was a hard guy." Mr. G hit a sharp liner to Dad at second base. The ball missed his glove and, once again, he took it right to the face. Dad was knocked unconscious, but the coach wasn't too concerned. He took Dad back to his house, but finding that his parents weren't home, he left him sprawled out on the front lawn. As Dad says, different times.

Academics, like athletics, came pretty easy for Dad, and he navigated his school years with relative ease. His sharp mind and quick sense of humor were evident early on, and it was, in fact, his humor that first appealed to Pam Pence (also known as my mom) when she met Dad through a friend. Mom remembers meeting Dad when she was sixteen and he was seventeen. "I truly believe he was in love with her since the day they met," Aunt Boo says. "Shortly after they started seeing each other, they had some kind of falling out. I remember seeing Mark sitting on the stairs of the house, talking to my mom, and he was crying. At the time I didn't know what it was about. I just remember standing there looking at him and thinking something terrible had happened because I had never seen him cry before." The breakup didn't last long, but their romance—now fifty-one years and counting—certainly has. In fact, they renewed their marriage vows in the spring of 2021.

The Pence household quickly became a second home for Mace, and he endeared himself to Pam's four brothers (the youngest of whom, Eric, was four) with goofy antics like pulling off the boys' dirty socks and trying to stuff them in their mouths. The kids loved him. At the Pence house, Mace had discovered a lightness of spirit not found in his own family home. He found himself hanging out there even when Pam was not at home.

Out on the playing fields of his youth, Mace dreamed of maybe someday playing for his beloved Detroit Tigers. Slugger Al Kaline was a favorite. In the same year that Dad graduated from Stevenson High in Livonia, his much-admired older brother was graduating from Albion College, about eighty miles to the west, where he had played basketball and baseball. Dad had always tagged along after his brother, and Greg's path sounded good to him, too. But Albion wasn't cheap and family finances were tight. He would need to work a year in order to save up enough money to start college the following fall. At various times that year, Dad held jobs laying carpet, working in an automotive plant, and even working in Detroit steel mills, where he'd stand inside massive boilers and use a jackhammer (held above his head) to remove carbon residue from the boiler walls. The jackhammer, he says, weighed more than he did. It was tough, dirty work, but it got him closer to his goal of attending college.

Dad's most lucrative job that year and for a few summers to follow was as a "gunite guy." He explains:

Gunite is essentially concrete that's blown through a big hose under high pressure and sticks to everything. So I was on a crew that used it to build swimming pools. It was a real tough job and they were real tough, badass guys who were doing the work. The first day of work, I showed up wearing my high school varsity jacket. They called me "College Boy" and made fun of me, then one guy blew gunite all over my varsity jacket.

Despite that first day's hazing, Mace stuck with the job and pretty quickly won over the rough and tumble crew. He traveled across the state with them, building swimming pools and, as he describes it, trying to distance himself from the trouble they courted. Petty, and sometimes not-so-petty, thievery seemed to be a favorite pastime of the pool-building crew. "I wonder to this day if any of those guys are still alive," Dad says. "I do know that several of them went to prison."

The gunite job was dangerous on more than one level, but the pay made it worth the risk. "I made a fortune as a gunite guy," Dad says. "At least it seemed like a fortune at the time. I made more than I could have at any other job."

But Albion College was still out of reach. He'd be headed to Michigan State in East Lansing instead. As Dad was a year ahead of Mom in school, they actually headed off to MSU together.

By that time, things had really started falling apart in the Macy home because of Dad's mom's drinking. Dad had no intention of ever returning to Livonia and says that as soon as the dorm doors opened his freshman year, he was gone for good.

Dad decided early on to pursue a law degree but settled on communications for his undergraduate degree reasoning that with an easier major he could carry a strong enough GPA to get into law school. (It worked. My dad is smart like that.) In the summers, he'd rejoin the gunite crew and squirrel away tuition money.

Meanwhile, Mom was pursuing a double major in social work and psychology. After graduating, she took a job in a residential treatment facility for developmentally delayed and emotionally disturbed young people. These were kids that couldn't be placed in foster care and for whom adoption wasn't really an option. It was emotionally taxing, but she loved it. (My mom is big-hearted like that.)

Mom and Dad both graduated in 1976 and would marry the following year. But they weren't done with school yet. Dad was accepted to the University of Detroit Law School and Mom began pursuing a master's degree in guidance and counseling at Michigan State. Both held down full-time jobs and attended classes in the evenings. By that time, Dad had traded in the gunite job for a desk gig. He hired on as an insurance claims adjuster. Here, once again, he was heeding his brother's advice and following in his footsteps. It was a good way for Mace to learn a little about the law without yet being able to practice, Greg reasoned. "I had to take a pay cut to go work for that insurance company," Dad recalls. But, on the plus side, there was considerably less chance of incarceration, not to mention the exposure to toxins inherent in the factory and swimming pool work he'd been doing.

Mace and Pam married in 1977, but before that date, a couple important events occurred. First, they took a driving trip out to Colorado, visiting Rocky Mountain National Park among other sites that left them awestruck. Mom had visited the Rockies on family trips with her parents, but it was Dad's first time seeing real mountains. For him, it was something like a movie come to life. A specific movie, actually.

A year or so earlier, he had seen the Robert Redford movie *Jeremiah Johnson*. "Pam and I watched it," Dad remembers. "Then I watched it again. And then again. And I thought, 'By God, I'm gonna be a mountain man. I'm going to the Rocky Mountains.'" After completing his law degree in 1980, that's just what he did. (Well, not exactly the mountain man part. He didn't trap any beaver or wrestle any bears. But he would, in the late 1980s and early '90s, win his age group in the Mountain Man Winter Triathlon five times, so that counts for something.) Incidentally, Mom was all in on the Colorado dream as well. "That first trip we took together really did plant a seed," she recalls, "that this would be a great place to live."

The other notable event that occurred before they got married occurred *right* before they got married. At that time, Michigan required blood tests to get a marriage license. Mom's test indicated that she had abnormal liver function. Mom recalls it as a "big surprise, but not too concerning." The diagnosis was autoimmune hepatitis—essentially, inflammation without a known cause.

When they were ready to have kids, Mom's doctors warned her that it would be high risk. But while I was a bit of a runt—4 pounds, 13 ounces—I was healthy. "Maybe more cautious people wouldn't have chosen to take that risk," Mom says. "But in general, we're not big worriers."

Still, it was pretty clear to Mom that it was asking a lot of her body to carry a child, especially as her liver function continued to worsen, so when my parents wanted to add a child to the family two years later, they made the decision to adopt a baby from Korea. Katelyn was six months old and adorable. Dad traveled to Korea to pick her up and remembers that on his flight home, seemingly every woman on the plane wanted a turn at holding her.

At the time I was born, my parents were living in a tiny rental house in Evergreen, a small, unincorporated town in the foothills about thirty minutes west of Denver. Money was tight in those years as Dad worked to establish his law practice. The guy who lived next door (George Wesley "Wes" Minard, the nicest mean-looking Harley rider you've ever seen) had a window-washing business, and Dad started helping out on weekends to make a few extra bucks. Wes knew that Dad, as a rock climber, wasn't worried about heights, so he had him do second-story windows. When they'd show up at a client's house, Wes loved to say, "This is my attorney, and he's here to help do the windows."

Living at the edge of the mountains, surrounded by a network of trails and dirt roads, Dad's fire for running was stoked. His runs got longer and he got stronger. He ran his first marathon (Denver) in 1984, the year after I was born. As he recounts the story, he took the whole thing pretty lightly and, several hours in, found himself disoriented and shivering uncontrollably in Washington Park. "I was bonking bad," Dad says, "but a woman gave me a donut and a blanket, and I started to recover." By the time he finished that marathon, he was already thinking about his next challenge. Hell, he was already a mountain man, why not an Ironman? The Ironman World Championship had captured the public's attention since its inception in 1978, and Dad couldn't resist. In 1986, he traveled to Kona to compete in the iconic event: 2.4-mile open-water swim, 112-mile bike ride across the lava desert, and a marathon run.

As Dad's athletic pursuits ramped up, the lawyering business was picking up too. He managed it all by lengthening his days. Something had to give, and that something was usually sleep. On weekdays, he'd set the alarm for 4:00 a.m., be out of the house by 4:30, and drive forty-five minutes to his Denver office in the dark. Over lunch, he'd run for an hour with two fellow Ironman participants. His business frequently took him out of the office, and Dad took advantage of the opportunity to add some variety to his training. If he needed to take a deposition in Grand Junction, he'd stop along the way and run up a favorite mesa trail. Over the years, he mentally compiled a map of favorite running routes across the state.

For many athletes, the Hawaii Ironman is a bucket list accomplishment. For Dad, it was more of a launch point (some might say "gateway drug") toward further adventures. In the mid-to-late 1980s, Dad and a small group of like-minded men and women would go on to pioneer the sport of ultra-running—that is, competing in trail and road races from 50k (31 miles) to beyond 100 miles, nonstop.

Dad's first foray into ultrarunning was another race that has taken on the luster of an American classic: the Leadville Trail 100 Run, aka the Race Across the Sky. Beginning and ending in Leadville, Colorado—America's highest incorporated city at 10,200 feet, the LT100 course is charted on rough roads and mountain trails and climbs and descends 15,600 feet, with elevations ranging from 9,200 to 12,620 feet. In most years, fewer than half the starters complete the race within the thirty-hour time limit. Today, the LT100 is on every serious ultrarunner's radar, but back in 1988 the race was still something of a novelty at only five years old. In fact, now that I think about it, the great race and I were born the same year!

Dad had never run anything longer than a marathon and was, it's fair to say, somewhat naïve about what a 100-miler at that altitude would require of body and mind. Runners attempting their first century race typically train for multiple years, gradually building up distances from marathon to 50k to 50 miles to 100k—all spaced out over many months. Dad had been running, swimming, cycling, and climbing consistently since the '86 Ironman, but honestly, this was an entirely different beast. Nothing pounds the body quite the way a 100-miler does. Factor in the high altitude and the lack of a sophisticated hydration and nutrition strategy, and, well, the chance for calamity was pretty high. Of course, Dad did have the X-factor on his side—his relentless positivity and an indomitable will to finish.

As a five-year-old kid, I had no idea what kind of challenge Dad had set for himself (and thank God for that or I would have been a nervous wreck). I was just excited to be in this honest-to-goodness mountain outpost, surrounded by cowboys and athletes and a crackling energy in the air that I had never felt in my life. All I knew was my dad was going to do something amazing—run a hundred miles without stopping!

The race began, as it always does, at 4:00 a.m. on a mid-August Saturday with a shotgun blast courtesy of race cofounder and Leadville local legend Ken Chlouber. A second blast thirty hours later—at 10:00 a.m. Sunday—marks the cutoff.

Along with roughly 250 other runners, Dad was off at the shot, provisioned only with two water bottles and a cheap flashlight he'd picked up at 7-Eleven on the drive to Leadville. Not exactly a state-of-the-art gear or hydration/ nutrition system.

The race is always held on the weekend before local

schools begin the fall term. Because my family had decamped to Leadville a few days before the race, I missed the back-to-school/meet-your-teacher open house held the Friday before the first day of school. Instead, on my first day of first grade, I would sheepishly walk into my classroom, and say, "Mrs. Jeffers, I'm the one who wasn't here on Friday, because I was at the Leadville 100 watching my dad." I had a great year with Mrs. Jeffers, who often let me work ahead on more advanced material. An anxious perfectionism was brewing within me. At the time, I had no idea that it would become one of my greatest powers and largest challenges.

I also didn't know at the time how important this event, this town, and this weekend would become to my family over the coming decades. My dad would go on to run and ride regularly in Leadville events, as would I. But the impact of that first race also set off something of a chain reaction through my family. At the time of this writing, seven members of my family have finished the 100-mile race. (My wife jokes that we'll never have to plan a family reunion as long as they keep holding the LT100.) Initially inspired by Dad's participation, my uncle Eric, my mom's youngest brother, has logged thirty-one consecutive LT100 starts (and finished twenty-six). Only two other runners in the race's history have run it more.

But back to 1988 and the run that started it all for the Macy/Pence clan. We'd planned to meet Dad at the race's halfway point, in a little ghost town called Winfield tucked deep in the mountains of the San Isabel National Forest.

Dad trotted in around 4:00 in the afternoon. It'd been twelve hours and he'd already run fifty miles. He looked and felt surprisingly good. In fact, he felt good enough about his split time and physical state that he decided to sit down on a blanket and have an impromptu picnic with us. This, I should point out, is not normal or advisable protocol for the middle of an ultraendurance race. But Mom and Dad are both exceptionally laid-back people. Mom told me later that looking back now, she didn't really grasp the enormity of what Dad was doing. "He was just out there having a good day," she says. And her breeziness was a reflection of Dad's own. "I was having a good time," Dad recalls. "I wasn't thinking about much of anything." He said he expected that he could run the second fifty miles in about the same time as the first, easily beating the thirty-hour cutoff. So we finished eating, and he was off, retracing his path on the way back to Leadville.

Of course, between Winfield and Leadville was another 8,000 feet of ascending and descending, including the nearly 3,000-foot climb back over Hope Pass, the race's highest point. By the time he reached the small town of Twin Lakes on the other side of Hope Pass at mile 60, Dad's body was starting to go into revolt. His quadriceps and hamstrings were so tight he could barely move. Pain shot through his feet with every step—he would later be diagnosed with stress fractures in the metatarsals of both feet. He was dehydrated and retching. And, of course, by then it was full dark.

Years later, when I asked him about it, he admitted that he'd blocked out a lot from that first race, but he remembers that at some point in the night, he hit bottom, physically and emotionally. "I was on my knees dry-heaving," Dad recalls. "It really did seem impossible."

The 7-Eleven flashlight had burned out after a couple hours, but in the dark, alongside his pacer, Cleve Schenk (comically and illogically wearing prescription sunglasses because he'd lost his normal glasses), he found a spark. "I told myself I would make it if I just kept moving. And as long as I kept moving, I kept believing it was possible."

While Dad was picking his way along the trail in the

dark, we were back at a motel in Leadville. Sometime around 4:00 a.m., Mom and my uncle Brian headed down to the finish line. The twenty-four-hour mark came and went. The twenty-five-hour mark—the cutoff to earn the larger commemorative belt buckle—likewise passed. But while other runners shuffled up 6th Street to be wrapped in hugs by elated (and relieved) friends and family, Dad still wasn't there. Mom and Uncle Brian drove out of town along the course and eventually found Dad a few miles away, still plugging along gamely after a very long night.

Meanwhile, friends from Evergreen had taken my sister and me to the finish line, where we waited. And waited. Patiently, as only sleep-deprived five- and three-year-olds can.

Being that age, we were blissfully unaware that Dad was in real danger now of missing the thirty-hour cutoff. But I do remember looking at that big, red digital clock off to the side of the finish line, ticking away the seconds, the minutes, the hours.

On the outskirts of town, Dad, Mom, and Uncle Brian were having a little bit of panic. It was nearing 10:00, and though Dad had no doubt his body could make the last couple of miles into town, they were having navigation problems. "I was trying to find Leadville!" Dad says. "I realized that the race was about to end, but I didn't know which way to go."

Mom recalls that the course wasn't marked, or not marked very well, and that by that point there were no other racers or race officials nearby to ask for directions. After a few confused minutes of hesitation—minutes that Dad truly could not spare—they did find the route into town. Mom and Uncle Brian headed back to town and left Dad to finish the race on his own.

I've witnessed and been personally involved in more race finishes than I can remember, but I know I'll never forget seeing Dad running up 6th Street toward the Leadville finish line in 1988. His body was wracked and his eyes were glazed. Nearly six hours into his second day of running, he was exhausted beyond comprehension. But when he saw my sister and me, he mustered a smile, scooped my sister up in his arms, and held my hand while he shuffled the final twenty meters to the finish.

One hundred thirty-five runners finished the Leadville Trail 100 that year. Dad finished 135th. His time of 29 hours, 56 minutes, 13 seconds was at that point the closest finish to the cutoff (in other words, the slowest recorded time or, colloquially, the "Last Ass Over the Pass") in the race's history. The fact that his time—after running for nearly thirty hours—came down to a mere 227 seconds under the wire, has made for a great story and a lot of laughs over the ensuing thirty-three years. But the serious truth is that that first Leadville Trail 100 set Dad's life on a new trajectory. Out there alone in the thin air, he'd learned what he was capable of. Dad had had a taste. And when the pain wore off and the stress fractures healed, he wanted more.

Watching him finish that race, through my five-year-old eyes, I had my own realization. My dad was Superman, and I wanted to be just like him.

In ensuing years, Dad would enter and finish Leadville four more times, bringing home the prestigious, gaudy belt buckle earned by racers who cross the line in less than twenty-five hours. More importantly, he finished strong in each of the next four attempts. He went in prepared and never made the mistake of underestimating the distance again.

Meanwhile, he broadened his ultraendurance experience

far beyond Leadville, seeking out and competing in some of the most challenging (and, yes, some would say, sadistic) races that like-minded athletes and organizers (often these people are one and the same) could dream up. Snowshoeing a hundred miles across Alaska? Sure. Running from the bottom of Death Valley to the top of Mount Whitney? Why not! A 155-mile jaunt across the Sahara? Fun run! Dad truly did get to experience the world and its cultures and people through these races, and in a way that you just can't if you're dropping in on a tourist junket. It's always been his favorite thing about these events.

As busy as his schedule was, Dad was nonetheless a constant presence in my life and in the life of my mom and sister, too. And that actually made him better than Superman, who disappears after he performs his heroic feats. Dad was there for the day-to-day stuff. In grade school I played soccer, baseball, and basketball. High school brought track and cross-country. Like his own father before him, Dad never missed a game or meet. I realize now that even more importantly, he was there for me emotionally. Dad and Mom were both completely committed to being engaged, available parents.

It's a funny thing about big races—you train and work, suffer, sweat, bleed, and obsess about them for months or even years in advance, and then... they're over, and the next day it's back to real life. The day after that first Leadville race, Dad went back to work; I started first grade; and Mom continued the vital role of keeping us all fed, clothed, and happy. But Mom was also in a race of her own. By the late 1980s her liver function was getting critical and she was placed on a transplant waiting list. She admits now that she was "pretty sick," but she carried on doing what needed to be done. "I guess this is just my personality," she says. "Yes, of course, I realized I could die, but I just didn't believe that was going to happen. I believed I would get a transplant and be okay."

In 1990, at age thirty-five, she was matched with a donor. After the procedure, her transplant surgeon told her that, given her preoperative condition, he was surprised she had still been functioning and not been confined to a hospital. Without the liver transplant, he went on to say, she'd likely had only another month and a half to live. Mom and Dad never made a big deal of that transplant. Now, as a parent myself, I'm sure they must have felt some anxiety about hypotheticals, but they really did take it in stride. My main memory of the period is fun at home with Uncle Brian while they were at the hospital. He took us to Jack in the Box, gave me a haircut on the deck, and taught me about race tactics in the road cycling peloton. Decades before #vanlife (or #anything) became a thing, Uncle B lived in his little red Subaru, delivering papers for a living and biking six hours a day. Back then I thought he was super cool. Now I know it.

Not long after her surgery, we all found ourselves in LA, where Mom competed in the Transplant Olympics, smoking the 5k that Dad and I ran as well. People who only know me through my racing and ultraendurance accomplishments usually assume that I get my toughness from my dad. They're half right.

TWO

*I've always loved Saturdays and today is Saturday,
and as is usual for me, I ran Evergreen Mountain,
which is near my house, and when I reached the
summit I had a conversation with my dad. My dad,
Jack Macy, died several years ago at age ninety-
three. We had a family gathering and spread his
ashes on the summit of Evergreen Mountain. I run
up there two or three times a week and I stop to
talk to him. Over the last couple of years I have
mentioned to him that I had concerns about my
cognitive function. Today, however, I told him I've
actually been diagnosed with ALZ disease, and it
made me cry. If he can actually hear and understand
what I've told him, he will be broken-hearted.*

*I always assumed I would live into my
nineties like my dad did. Now I'm not so sure
that's likely to happen, and that makes me cry as
well. The good news is I have my family to help
me through this process, whatever it may be, and
perhaps most significantly young Dr. Sawyer.
Hopefully, he can pull the irons out of the fire.
And finally, I have to quit this crying stuff.*

—MACE'S JOURNAL

WHEN I WAS TEN OR ELEVEN, my Dad's law firm instituted
a policy allowing partners to take a one-time three-month
sabbatical. Mom and Dad jumped all over it. (It's good

they did, too, because the firm rescinded the policy short-ly thereafter.) For Dad, there was no question where they'd go: to the Last Frontier! Jagged mountains, untamed rivers, massive glaciers, animals that might eat you (most fear-some, we would discover, were the mosquitoes)—Alaska had everything a wannabe Jeremiah Johnson could ask for. My parents bought an old Airstream travel trailer for $7,000 and locked up the house, and in the summer of 1994 we hit the road north. I made it all the way to the outskirts of Denver before excitedly calling a friend from a truck stop pay phone to tell him how far we'd driven. We only had 3,000+ miles still to go. So, yeah, I was excited too.

Three months in Alaska! In the weeks before we left, I had friends over for sleepovers in the camper parked in our driveway. My eleven-year-old head swam with images of snow, sled dogs, bears, eagles, and moose, but mostly fish, specifically wild salmon. Many successful endurance athletes have—for better or worse—a natural tendency to hyperfo-cus on the obsession of the moment. Sure, I wasn't yet an endurance athlete in 1994, but the predilections were already forming, and my hyperfocus had locked in on salmon fishing.

The drive in itself—all ten days of it—was a grand adven-ture and a prolonged exercise in goofiness. We quickly dis-covered a kind of "road warrior" brotherhood among fellow Airstream owners. As we passed other Airstreams on the road or encountered them in RV campgrounds, we became aware of the Wally Byam Caravan Club, named after Airstream's founder. We christened our own rig "The Wally" and started flashing the "secret" signal to every Airstream driver we passed. The secret signal—the "hang loose" shaka sign—was, incidentally, entirely our own contribution to Wally culture. We giggled and hooted our way along the ALCAN highway (the roughly 1,500-mile route that connects Alaska to the contiguous US, across Canada), delighting in the confused looks or, occasionally, the awkward reciprocal shaka, we received in reply. Many club members sported his-and-hers matching Pilot and Co-Pilot hats, jackets, and/or one-piece coveralls. I thought that stuff was *so* geeky at the time (but who knows how Amy and I will be dressed when we hit the road like that in a couple decades). The entire route is now paved, but back in '94 it was still notorious for its rough, unpaved sections. I remember a lot of bumps, dust, and traffic jams. (Lots of opportunities to flash that Wally sign!)

Most of our fellow pilgrims on the ALCAN seemed to be retirees. We were on a different, family-centric schedule and were usually the last ones to roll into a campground at night and several hours behind the last ones to leave the next day. Lots of the campgrounds had access to lakes or streams, so I got to fish my way across Canada. I didn't have much luck, but it served to stoke my ever-growing desire for the king salmon I coveted.

Looking back, a few memories from that trip remain prominent. First, mosquitoes. They were legion and large. I mean, they were monsters. I remember fishing with a head net on, trying to maintain concentration as the bloodsuckers carried out a sustained multifront assault against the mesh. One night, at a campground called Willow Creek just north of Anchorage, the assassins somehow managed to breach the Wally's perimeter. They came in waves—we surmised later that it was through a sink drain—and mercilessly attacked any exposed flesh. The story has become family lore most notably for the fact that it is the one time anyone can remember my easy-going dad losing his cool. I mean, *really* losing it. "He was like Jack Nicholson in *The Shining*," remembers Mom, laughing. "He was flailing away with a magazine in one hand, and spraying anything that moved with repellent in the other."

Surveying the carnage the next morning, I was oblivious. I had slept through the whole thing. Meanwhile, Katelyn had one skinny arm completely covered in angry red welts. It had been out of the sleeping bag and an easy target.

Meanwhile, I kept fishing. It was high summer in Alaska, the land of the midnight sun, and my parents would let me fish until one or two in the morning if I wanted. No king salmon yet, but I was undaunted. Later in the trip, one of Dad's best friends from college, Ed Sandifer, flew up from Michigan to meet us. One day, Dad hired a guide to take us out on the Kenai River—famous for salmon runs that can number more than a million fish. I suspect that Dad and Ed had agreed ahead of time that whichever of them hooked a fish first would let me land it, and that's just what Ed did. But at the moment Ed handed his rod to me, neither of us knew just what was on the end of the line. It turned out to be a 40-pound king. I guess I outweighed it, but not by much. I reeled it in and in doing so pretty much checked off the entirety of my summer to-do list. It was the greatest accomplishment in my life to that point in time (and maybe still in the top ten or so).

Another memorable stop along the way was Talkeetna, the quirky little town a couple hours north of Anchorage that inspired the town of Cicely in the '90s TV series *Northern Exposure* and serves as a staging point for mountaineering treks up nearby Denali. We didn't attempt to summit Denali but did happen to be in town for the annual Moose Dropping Festival, where Dad and I had a blast running a 5k race together. Later in the trip, we got to visit the kennels of legendary Iditarod musher Martin Buser, where my sister and I fell in love with sled dog puppies. Sadly, they were not available for adoption.

One more indelible memory from the trip was a

chartered halibut fishing excursion that went frighteningly wrong. Dad had saved a few bucks by booking us on the cheapest fishing charter at the marina, and we found ourselves on a crappy old Chris-Craft boat with a newly married couple and Captain Dow, a rangy old guy who reeked of alcohol and sported a big scar from ear to mouth that might have been called "unsightly" away from Alaska. On the way out to sea, he told me about "the good old days when we used to shoot bears from bush planes with machine guns." Far from shore, the boat caught fire. I remember one of the passengers yelling, "Abandon ship! Abandon ship!" to which Dad replied, "Abandon ship, bullshit! We're miles from shore!" Fortunately, Dad and Dow, whose hangover seemed to be wearing off, were able to put the fire out together, and we made it back to the Wally safe and sound. Once again, my own father had proven himself Superman—at least in my eyes. It made for a great true-adventure story to tell my friends back home in Evergreen.

As I write this, my own two children are eleven and nine—the same age as my sister and me at the time of our Alaskan adventure. I honestly can't imagine what it would be like to have three months truly away, camping every night with no phones, no TV, no tech—virtually no connection to the wider world. And if I'm being perfectly honest with myself, I'm not entirely sure I could handle it, but it's pretty wild to think about.

Mom received her liver transplant in 1990, four years before our Alaskan summer. Over the years leading up to that—ever since adopting Katelyn, in fact—Mom had had a growing desire to give something back in exchange for the gift that was my sister. Katelyn had spent the first three months of her life in an orphanage and the next three in a foster home.

"When Mace was in Korea picking up Katelyn, he had a chance to spend some time with the woman who was fostering her," Mom recalls. "When he came back he said it was really obvious how much this woman loved Katelyn and that she had taken such good care of her. So I always had this in my head that I wanted to do that for another child someday, to get them off to a good start. Those early months of a child's life are so important. I knew I couldn't do it leading up to my liver transplant, but during that summer in Alaska, I just got the feeling it was the right time. I talked to Mace about it, and it wasn't like he was jumping up and down about it, but he was certainly agreeable to the idea of having one baby for three months, and that's really all I anticipated doing."

Shortly after Mom and Dad applied to be foster parents and went through the vetting process, they were matched with a baby; the plan was for a short-term placement with a single child while his or her parent(s) could get things back together. But as it turns out, the baby, Donavahn, had a four-year-old half-sister, Haven. Though this was considerably more than what they had signed up for, there was no way my parents were going to split them up. I remember my sister and I being excited to have these kids join our family for a few months—especially the baby.

Three months came and went, but with no positive placement options for Donavahn and Haven, they stayed on with us. What's more, my parents were soon informed that Haven had a biological brother, Keegan, who at nine years old was two years younger than I, so they took him in too. This was all meant to be on a temporary basis, but anyone who has had experience in the fostering world knows that situations are often fluid and not typically very tidy. To make the long (still ongoing, actually) story short, my parents went on to adopt Donavahn at age two and continued providing foster care for Haven and Keegan, as their needs and situations required, throughout their growing up years.

Dad and I have particularly fond memories of a trip to Moab, Utah, that we shared with Keegan. Keeg and I were probably fourteen and sixteen, and Dad had been invited by his adventure-racing teammate, Isaac Wilson, to work as a volunteer instructor at a three-day Adventure-racing camp. Keeg kept saying things like, "Mace, you and your friends are all totally crazy!" when it was time for a new activity like camping, mountain biking, or rappelling. Nonetheless, he persevered and completed every discipline along with me and the adult participants, thanks largely to encouragement and support from Dad and Rebecca Rusch (who was also a guide at the camp and would later become a legendary mountain biker by winning the Leadville 100 four times).

As a kid playing baseball on the street in Livonia, Michigan, my dad imagined himself as the 1960s Detroit Tigers slugger Al Kaline. Through my own grade school years, I followed the exploits of superstars like Michael "Air" Jordan, Bo "Knows" Jackson, and "Neon" Deion Sanders, but in truth, I identified more with the scrappy, overachieving role players like Dennis Rodman (though not his look) and Steve Kerr.

Of course, I also cheered for our local Colorado sports standouts like Nuggets star Dikembe Mutombo and Rockies Dante Bichette, Eric Young, and Larry Walker. I emulated these guys on the playground just like the rest of my classmates at Wilmot Elementary. But, largely because of my dad, I had other athletic heroes too—ones not known to many of my classmates. For as far back as my memory goes, Dad and I have always watched the Tour de France on TV, and I knew the names of all the top riders. Because of Dad, I also came to understand the intricacies and strategies of team cycling. American Greg LeMond, who had won the race in 1986, '89, and '90, was an early hero of mine, but I admired his rivals, like Frenchmen Laurent Fignon and Bernard Hinault, too. And I was pumped about the American mountain bikers of the era like Ned Overend, Mike Kloser, John Tomac, and Tinker Juarez. To keep my little legs pumping on our rides up the hills near our home, Dad would adopt a British accent and do a spot-on imitation of the incomparable Tour announcer Phil Liggett:

"It's Fignon, LeMond, and Hinault, side by side!... Hinault takes the lead, but here comes LeMond! He's pulling away. It's... LeMond! He wins the stage at the line. What a finish!"

I would thrust my hands skyward, blowing kisses to imaginary crowds. Dad would imitate crowd noises through laughter and we'd peddle on through the Colorado sunshine. Dad always had a way to make physical exertion fun.

I was an athlete for all seasons in high school, competing in cross-country and soccer in the fall, basketball in the winter, and track in the spring. (Evergreen High, like many mountain west schools, now has a mountain bike team but didn't yet in the '90s.) I loved competing in all sports, and I guess I was something of a natural athlete, but I was also the kind of kid that pushed himself to work beyond those natural abilities. This was perhaps most obvious in basketball. I was skinny (5'10", 135 lbs.) with mediocre talent, but I was always the one diving for loose balls and harassing the other team with relentless defense. Scrappy and intense, that was me... Rodman sans attitude and tats. That intensity also translated to track and cross-country, and I made All-State in both those sports, but my best times weren't quite impressive enough to get any notice from major college programs.

While I was pushing myself in various high school sports, Dad was continuing to raise the bar on his own athletic pursuits. After collecting five sub-thirty-hour Leadville Trail 100 belt buckles, he began looking for different challenges. Not surprisingly, the call of the wild drew him back to Alaska. The year after our family trip, Dad returned in 1995 to participate in the annual Iditasport human-powered ultrarace. The race had evolved a bit since its founding in the early 1980s, but it's essentially a 100-mile race on the same course as the historic Iditarod dogsled race, but instead of dogsleds, participants used either Nordic skis, running shoes, snowshoes, or bicycles to navigate the course, pulling their own emergency supply sled behind them. Dad chose to run the course in snowshoes. He finished third in 1995 and went on to win the race three times from '96 to '99. He also won his age group in the World Snowshoe Championship (held in Colorado) in 1996. It may have been the sort of "world championship" that goes unknown beyond the state line, but as Dad always says, "You beat everyone who's too scared to show up, Bud." And there was probably truth to that since that particular race involved snowshoeing up and down Mt. Elbert, Colorado's highest peak at 14,439 feet.

I remember Dad coming home from that first Alaskan snowshoe race in 1995 with a participant T-shirt. On the back was printed a rough rendering of the course—I guess you could use it as a map if you got lost, and getting lost was a real danger in this race. On the front was printed the race's rather ominous but refreshingly honest slogan: "COWARDS WON'T SHOW AND THE WEAK WILL DIE!"

Thankfully, Dad always came back, and he always came back with stories. One year, he did get lost in a severe snowstorm, unable to find anyone else on the course (if he was even on the course) except for a group of rowdy and "drunk as shit" Alaskan snowmobilers who could not understand what a middle-aged guy in running tights was doing pulling a sled across the tundra in -30° temperatures. He eventually found his way—and subsequently found out that the rest of the pack, including racers and media, had been following his meandering tracks all the way. I remember dinner gatherings with friends where Dad would hold court, captivating everyone with such stories—mostly true, but maybe augmented with a little hyperbole and always with great humor and colorful language (various shades of blue). Dad was a raconteur. And as I listened to him tell these tales of adventure, I imagined myself with him, out there challenging the elements, my imagination sweeping me a long way from the high school gyms and running ovals of Jefferson County.

The only thing Dad liked to do as much as run in the snow was run through the desert, so in 1995, when he was asked by a fellow ultraathlete to serve as a last-minute fill-in for a team member in the inaugural Eco-Challenge in Moab, Utah, he didn't hesitate. The fact that he didn't really know what the Eco-Challenge was didn't affect his decision in the least.

The Eco-Challenge circa 1995, brainchild of future "super" producer Mark Burnett (*Survivor, The Apprentice,* etc.), was a multisport, multiday adventure race modeled after the Raid Gauloises, an expedition/adventure race first held in New Zealand in 1989. The Eco-Challenge—staged in the desolate deserts and canyonlands of southern Utah—introduced extreme multiday adventure racing to the US. The fellow ultraathlete who had invited Dad to join his team was Marshall Ulrich, who would quickly become one of Dad's closest friends and by anyone's standards is now a legendary figure in the endurance racing world.

Prior to that, Dad had competed in a handful of

twelve-hour-to-twenty-four-hour adventure races and loved the variety of disciplines that usually included some combination of rock climbing; biking; running; and a water sport like swimming, kayaking, or rafting. These races also involved navigating a course with map and compass.

The Eco-Challenge in Utah was broadcast that year on MTV and later on the Discovery Channel and USA Network. I've heard both Dad and Marshall tell stories of that first Eco-Challenge, and the main takeaway is that they were competent in the various athletic disciplines; pretty much a disaster at navigating the course; and, most importantly, had a blast and forged what would become a lifelong friendship. Regarding the navigational strategies, Dad recalls that when they found themselves at a loss, he would climb one sandstone spire and Marshall would climb another, and then they would both scan the horizon and shout out to the other if they saw any racers from another team. If they did, they'd scramble down and try to regain the course until they got lost again. Not surprisingly, they didn't win that first Eco-Challenge, but they did finish, even after the other three members of their team dropped out. In fact, as fate would have it, they formed a new team during that race. As Marshall recalls, he and Dad were making their way from one canyon (the wrong one) to another (the one where they were supposed to be) when they encountered the remnants of another depleted team, Bob Haugh and Lisa Smith-Batchen. Bob Haugh remembers the auspicious meeting well. "This was day three or four of the race and we were seeing all this misery out there... people sitting on the side of the trial, some crying, and everybody dejected. We ran into Mark and Marshall smack in the middle of this slot canyon, and they were the first people I'd seen in days that were smiling. I'd never seen these guys before, but they were just moving along and having a good time."

The four strays decided to finish the race together, and a new team, shortly thereafter christened the Stray Dogs, was born. That team (with a few rotating members throughout the years) would become a fixture in every Eco-Challenge to follow. Marshall memorialized many of the "Dogs'" misadventures in his 2011 memoir, *Running on Empty*. After recounting a story about getting lost during an Eco-Challenge in Malaysian Borneo, he wrote: "Some of the inexperienced teams had thought (wrongly) that because we were Eco-Challenge veterans, they should follow us. (One of the Stray Dogs' trademark navigational tactics is getting completely lost and laughing our asses off about it.)"

Wow, what a year 1995 must've been for Dad. Let's see: that's the Iditasport 100-mile snowshoe race in Alaska in February, the Leadville Trail 100 at high altitude in his home state of Colorado in August, and in April the Eco-Challenge—a 350-mile race across Utah comprised of running, hiking, horseback riding, mountain biking, climbing, rafting, canyoneering, and canoeing. Oh, and there was the usual mix of triathlons and snowshoe races thrown in to boot. Not to mention nearly nightly bike rides up the mountains in our backyard with me. Then there were the new foster kids... and, oh yeah, sixty-hour workweeks as an attorney. I honestly don't know how he did it.

But of all those races, it was the Eco-Challenge that really grabbed hold of Dad. It was the "adventure" part of adventure racing that did it. He loved being out there battling nature and throwing everything he had at the variety of challenges such races offered up. "Adventure racing," says Dad, "changed everything for me. There's just more to it, and it's taken me all over the world." He's not exaggerating. The eight Eco-Challenges he competed in from 1995 to 2002 were held in Utah, Canada, Australia, Morocco, Argentina and Chile, Borneo, New Zealand, and Fiji.

Hearing about Dad's adventures—even watching them on TV—never got old. I didn't get to travel to the exotic locations of the Eco-Challenges, but I experienced them vicariously through Dad. And then when the races would finally air after months of anxious waiting, we'd record them on VHS and watch them again in the evenings while lifting weights together in the basement.

Sometimes Dad brought home more than just memories and colorful stories. My senior year in high school, the Eco-Challenge was in Borneo, where day after day of soggy jungle trekking, spelunking, and river swimming left about half of the racers with leptospirosis, a disease that causes flu-like symptoms, vomiting, and diarrhea and can result in serious damage to the liver, kidneys, and lungs. Dad made it home before the symptoms really kicked in, but on the way home from his first day back to work, he found himself shivering uncontrollably with fever and muscle spasms. He'd pulled the vehicle onto the shoulder of I-70, unable to drive safely. He's never been a techie, but for some reason he was an early adopter of the cell phone (at that time what we called a "truck phone" that mounted in the vehicle and was as big as a briefcase), so he called Mom for a ride to the hospital. I remember him at my basketball games months later, still on crutches due to ongoing muscle cramps. I'll state the obvious now, in case the reader is wondering: adventure racing is, well, a different kind of fun that appeals to a different kind of person. Still, by the time I was eighteen, I'd pretty much decided that, like Dad, I was that kind of person.

Leading up to my high school graduation I wasn't really sure where I wanted to go to school and whether I'd pursue running or triathlon, but when Dad offered to take me on a postgraduation trip, I immediately knew where I wanted to go. A few days after graduation in 2001, Dad and I flew to Anchorage, where we rented a pickup truck with an old camper on the back. We didn't really have an agenda other than exploring wild places (while running), catching fish, and—oh, yeah—trying to figure out my future.

Dad and I relished a run up and down the 4,826-foot Mt. Marathon, which rises steeply from the sea near Seward. A legendary place in the mountain running world because of its annual 4th of July race ("the toughest 5k on the planet" according to *Outside* magazine and one of the oldest foot races in America), Mt. Marathon proved even more impressive in person. I loved running up that thing next to my dad, and I was beginning to think experiences like this would need to play a big role in my adult life. Our camaraderie was seamless and natural; at nearly fifty, Dad was young, fun, sharp, fit, and vibrant. As usual, he had all the answers.

I found an answer about my future in a book I'd brought along for the trip. I'd stay up late under the midnight sun reading *Running with the Buffaloes*, Chris Lear's chronicle of a year spent with the distance runners at the University of Colorado at Boulder. The book followed the struggles of unheralded walk-ons who became All-Americans through perseverance and hard work. I decided that this would be my path too. Dad agreed, and we created a plan for my next step in life.

I was accepted to CU and spent the rest of the summer training while also working for Wes's window washing company (yup, I even followed Dad's footsteps into that short-lived career, which paid a pretty good hourly rate and allowed me to practice navigating city streets). A week after the fall semester began, the walk-on contenders for the cross-country team would compete in a tryout race. The top three finishers

would win a spot on the team. Inspired by Mom's perseverance through kidney failure, I raced hard at the tryout, continuing forward after a midstride vomit on the final hill to
finish first among the prospective walk-ons. First to congrat-
ulate me: Dad. I was indeed going to run with the Buffaloes.

THREE

*Today I had a rather typical training run up
Evergreen Mountain, when I came across four
twenty-something-year-olds on mountain bikes
ahead of me. I picked up the speed and passed one
of these young men before he reached the summit.*

*When I reached the summit, I sat down as
I often do where we scattered my dad's ashes,
to think of Dad and Mom for a moment before
returning down the hill. As I sat on the summit, the
young men passed behind me on their mountain
bikes and one of them called out to his friends, "I
want to be just like that guy when I get older."*

*When I heard that I thought about telling
them I had just been diagnosed with ALZ disease.
I didn't do that because I didn't want to interfere
and potentially ruin their nice fall afternoon.*

—Mace's Journal

WHILE I WAS RUNNING with the Buffaloes in my freshman
and sophomore years at CU, Dad continued to compete with
the Stray Dogs in Eco-Challenges: 2001 took them to New
Zealand and 2002 to Fiji. The latter, Dad would say, was the
toughest of eight Ecos he had done up to that time—and his
favorite, naturally. Unfortunately, it would also turn out to
be the last Eco for a long time. Eco-Challenge producer Mark
Burnett's reality TV show *Survivor* (he served as co–executive producer) had debuted in the spring of 2000 and became

a smash hit. Burnett would follow that up with a string of other winners including *The Apprentice, The Contender, Shark Tank,* and *The Voice.* While the Eco-Challenge was on ice, other high-profile (though not as commercially successful) adventure races filled the void. Most notable of these were the World Championship and the Primal Quest, which debuted in Telluride, Colorado, in 2002.

After two years of running cross-country (along with track) at CU, I came to the realization that I wasn't quite of the caliber to race with the Olympic-level runners in coach Mark Wetmore's program. It had been an incredibly rewarding experience, but I was ready for something else. As a kid, I had watched my dad evolve from a marathon runner into an ultrarunner, then a triathlete and adventure racer. There was just so much to do out there—the more out there, the better.

I entered my first adventure race in 2003, after my sophomore year. It was a two-man, twenty-four-hour event in Utah's Wasatch Mountains. Despite floundering in the paddling segment of the event, my teammate, Mark Falender, and I made up enough time in the running, cycling, and fixed rope segments to finish second in the field of around fifty teams. We were stoked... and I was hooked, just as Dad had been after his first Eco-Challenge eight years earlier. Other twelve- and twenty-four-hour multidiscipline races in Colorado and Utah followed. I sometimes competed as part of a two-person team and sometimes solo. Dad and I often both participated in these races, but never on the same team. By this time, our athletic arcs had already intersected and begun to diverge. I had surpassed him in most sports. (Snowshoe racing was probably the last one where he retained an edge, though we had also diverged there when I was in high school.) There was never a dramatic passing of the torch or a cinematic moment where the student became the master or anything like that. It just happened naturally, and Dad supported me every way he could. He crewed countless races of mine over the years, driving to remote aid stations to provide food, water, clothing, and encouragement, but the real edge he gave me was those affirmations he implanted deep in my brain going all the way back to my toddler years: "Keep hammering, Bud!"... "Don't quit."... "I believe in you."

With Dad, it was never overbearing, never emotionally freighted with anything but love and belief—even when the stakes were a lot higher than the top of the hills we'd pedal up behind our house when I was a kid. I've read a lot of athlete memoirs over the years and there's a pretty common thread to a lot of high-achiever backstories—that of the domineering parent, one who perhaps is looking to vicariously relive his or her own glories—or atone for failures—through their child. In deference to that tried-and-true narrative motif, I'll take this opportunity to relay a brief moment when Dad and I had our own charged conflict. The setting was Glenwood Springs, Colorado, and the event, the Endurance Challenge at Sunlight, a twelve-hour ski mountaineering race in 2008. The race began at 6:00 a.m. and ended at 6:00 p.m., and the goal was to do as many laps as possible, ascending the ski mountain using climbing skins and then alpine skiing back down. I would end up gaining 28,500 vertical feet within that time span. Dad was crewing for me, which meant he was responsible for making sure I was getting the right hydration, nutrition, clothing, and lights at the right intervals as I came through the feed zone at the bottom. Before the race, I had meticulously calculated calorie burn and scheduled my ingestion accordingly—this energy gel at this time, that bar at that time, etc. Dad's job was to give each to me at the right time, and I helped him out by scrawling notes on a piece of paper early that morning. They made complete sense to me, and I figured they would to Dad as well because his penmanship is actually worse than mine, which is a rare talent.

Knowing that I'd probably be ready for a boost down the homestretch, I noted some caffeinated gels to be handed out only in the final three hours of the race. But Dad errantly delivered them several hours before schedule. I ate one without realizing the mistake and copped my caffeine buzz (and inevitable subsequent crash) much earlier than planned. I was livid. After I realized the mistake, I unloaded on Dad on the next lap. "Dad, I wrote down that I only wanted the caffeinated gels later on! Come on!" I skied off in a blind rage. Thirty seconds later I felt about ten inches tall. How could I yell at the man who never failed me, who never showed me anything but love and support, who—no matter how hard we were grinding—had always managed to keep it fun and keep things in perspective? Plus, he had driven me all the way here, paid for our hotel room, and was about to spend a full day standing in the cold so I could grab a gel and a bottle every couple of hours. That wasn't who I was.

At our next scheduled meet-up, I apologized through tears. Dad graciously laughed it off.

And that's it. That was our *Great Santini* moment. Our version of, "I hate you! I didn't ask to be born!" Only ours was, "I love you. I'm sorry I stupidly yelled at you."

Back in my junior year I had joined the CU Club Triathlon Team, finishing tenth in the 2004 Collegiate National Championship at Olympic distance (1,500-meter swim, 40-kilometer bike, 10-kilometer run). During this time I also started entering mountain bike races. For me, this was a natural. I'd been grinding up (and flying down) mountain roads and trails around our house since I was five. When I got a little older—twelve or thirteen—a favorite ride was up Bergen Peak in Evergreen. I vividly recall riding to the trailhead with my friend Alex Dobbs, stripping off our shirts, stashing them in the bushes, and happily cranking up the single-track trail. No food, no water, on bikes that wouldn't qualify as anywhere near trail-worthy by today's standards. It made no difference to us. When we topped out after about five miles and 2,000 vertical feet to an elevation of 9,701', the hard part lay ahead: coming back down on no-suspension, rim-brake bikes that, as hand-me-downs from our dads, were way too big for us. Somehow we made it down alive, and we spent the next couple hours at the Pizza Hut buffet, back to work as hungry, awkward kids trying to look cool for the girls.

Bike technology had progressed considerably by the time I reached my early twenties and competed in rides like 24 Hours of Moab, which was, as the name implies, a mountain bike race in which athletes ride as many loops as they can on a technical trail nonstop through an entire day and night.

I ought to mention that I was still fully engaged in academics at CU. I began college on a premed track, largely inspired by the lifesaving work of the doctors who had performed my mom's liver transplant. I loved science, particularly anatomy and physiology, and the anticipated workload of medical school didn't intimidate me. I pushed hard enough in organic chemistry to earn the highest score on the final exam out of hundreds of students, but I was also discovering (not for the first time) the potential costs of single-minded dedication to a goal. Yes, I was killing it in academics and athletics, but that left very little time for socializing, relationships, and the rest of life.

That's about when I met Amy, a fellow Colorado native

a year ahead of me at CU. She was (and remains!) a smart, funny woman whose humor and spirit seemed to have a magical way of cracking through my innate intensity. She bought me a beer on our first date because, at twenty, I was still underage. As Amy and I grew together and I thought more about life after college, I realized med school probably wouldn't fit well with my aspirations for adventure racing, travel, and family. But teaching might.

Back in Evergreen, Mom's health was starting to fail again. She had contracted hepatitis C from a blood transfusion she had received during her liver transplant twelve years earlier. From 2000 to 2002 she fought the disease through her relentless drive and an equally aggressive medical protocol. The meds finally mitigated hepatitis, but they, along with the disease itself and her ongoing immunosuppressant drugs for the liver transplant, had ruined her kidneys. So in 2002, Mom received a new kidney from her brother, my uncle Brian—the same uncle who had cared for and entertained my sister and me when Mom had undergone her liver transplant back when I was seven years old. She couldn't have conjured up a better donor. Brian Pence was, like my dad and his own younger brother, Eric, a model of good health and habits as well as an ultrarunner and avid mountain biker. To everyone reading this, a little free advice: be nice to your siblings—you may need spare parts someday.

In the fall of my junior year at CU, I got my first big opportunity as an adventure racer when I was invited to race Adventure Xstream Expedition Moab. I wrote about this race in some detail in *The Ultra Mindset* so I won't rehash all the details here, but to sum up the experience: I raced with a top team of experienced pros; Dad crewed for us (as usual); we battled hard against a tough field including a top-notch team from Crested Butte, CO; I held my own in a race that included trekking, mountain biking, kayaking, and fixed ropes, and we won the race and the $8,000 first prize (split four ways). Not a bad beginning! An extra couple thousand dollars doesn't seem like that much to me these days as I enter my forties, but at the time it was huge.

As my undergraduate career at CU wound down, my adventure racing career—well, that's probably an overly impressive word for it—let's say my AR "experiences" kept growing. In January of my senior year, I traveled to Mexico to compete in my first international adventure race, Extreme Adventure Hidalgo. Most notable for me was that this was the first time I'd teamed up with Dave Mackey and Danelle Ballengee, two super-experienced, elite endurance athletes I had grown up admiring. Another athlete I admired, Dad, was with us too, competing with his own three-man team.

I was invited to join a different pro team, Team SOLE (sponsored by a custom orthotic company), for the Explore Sweden Adventure Race a few months later. It was one extreme (sunbaked desert, extreme heat, rugged canyons, slickrock, and mountains of Moab and Mexico) to the other (bitter cold, vast glaciers, ice-choked rivers, and blizzard conditions of northern Sweden). The competition in Sweden was definitely world-class, as was the level of suffering. Each race tested me. Each took me near the brink of collapse or quitting, but in each I was buoyed by an inner resolve to keep pushing. Dad's mental training sustained me at my lowest points, as did his presence as a crew member in Moab. Our team missed the podium in Sweden, but we persevered through brutal conditions that forced some of the toughest racers in the world to call it quits. We finished sixth. "Sixth" is the least-important word in that sentence. Plus I had gotten to race with and learn from legendary athletes who would become my friends and colleagues: my teammates, Paul Romero, Karen Lundgren, and Darren Clarke; world champion Mike Kloser and his teammates; renowned adventure racer and mountain biker Rebecca Rusch; and more. They were all so cool and tough and accomplished, but in the hierarchy of my mind none held a candle to Dad.

Amy had taken a teaching job at Denver Academy after graduating, and when I graduated a year later, I was offered a job at the same independent private school. It would have been a good, solid job promising clear career progression—a logical choice. I decided to pursue adventure racing instead. Potential income depended upon sponsorships (of which I had none) and prize money. To that point in time, my total earnings in races had been just a few thousand dollars plus some free gear and travel. But I believed in myself, and my parents and Amy encouraged me to go for it. I was twenty-two. Honestly, what better time to fully commit to the rigors of training, traveling, and competing in a sport with just a bit of earning potential than when I was young, healthy, unmarried, and already broke?

I competed in two more expedition races with Team SOLE, the same crew from Explore Sweden. EcoMotion Pro in Brazil was five days of slogging through mud and rain that ended with a nonpodium (read: no prize money) finish. We did better in the Desafio de los Volcanes, an expedition race in Patagonia. The race started on a beach in southern Chile and continued across the country to San Martin de los Andes, a beautiful mountain town in Argentina. Second place got us a check, but I can't remember the unremarkable amount—though I do remember a zero balance in my bank account around that time. My racing was taking me to some of the most breathtaking places in the world, but I could barely afford to eat.

For some time I had been talking with my Extreme Adventure Hidalgo teammates Dave Mackey and Danelle Ballengee about forming a team that could attract sponsors. Fortunately, in late 2005, we secured a deal with the skiwear company Spyder. I was paid $1,250 per month (which seemed like just about enough at the time), and Spyder committed to funding our team to adventure race around the world. At twenty-two years old, I could legitimately call myself a professional adventure racing athlete, and better yet, I was part of a team that had the talent and experience to compete against the best in the world.

The next four years would see the highs and lows to be expected from any athletic endeavor: a win at the 2006 Raid World Series in Australia with Team Spyder; another Swedish "sufferfest" (though this time in the summer) at the 2006 Adventure Racing World Championship, where a navigational lapse—largely my fault—likely cost us a podium finish; a shattered clavicle in a Moab mountain bike race that caused me to miss Primal Quest 2006. I learned to navigate courses across deserts, jungles, mountains, and tundra, while also navigating the psychological highs and lows of this somewhat fringe athletic avocation I'd chosen to pursue. Along the way, I continued to acquire the layers of experience and grit necessary to stay in the race. That's another lesson I learned from watching Dad. He didn't win a ton of the races he entered, but he always finished. Amy and I spent about nine months in New Zealand, where we lived primarily in a car and I focused on adventure racing. That life was good and simple, and the company was great—both Amy and the down-to-earth Kiwis we befriended. My paddling skills improved significantly, and I completed the Coast to Coast, a legendary one-day run-bike-run-bike-kayak-bike race across the South Island.

Despite pretty consistent successes, adventure racing was still a marginal living at best. In between training and competing, I'd pick up substitute teaching shifts or work in hospitality personnel services (corporatespeak for serving food and busing tables) at a country club in Evergreen where Katelyn worked. Even when I appeared with Dad on the cover of *Adventure Sports* magazine in 2005, staying humble wasn't a problem.

By 2007, it was obvious that my cobbled-together employment schedule wasn't enough. I accepted a job teaching English at the same private high school where Amy taught. I enjoyed teaching from the start and was energized by the prospect of impacting students' lives in the same way that certain teachers and coaches had impacted mine. Soon after, I began working toward a master's degree in education and began thinking about eventually entering academic administration. Even while working full-time, I reasoned that with summers off—and by training like a maniac on weekends and off-hours—I could still manage to compete at a high level.

As it turns out, I gained employment as a teacher in Jefferson County, Colorado, just in time to have my already meager salary frozen due to the global financial crisis of 2007–2008. But I suppose it could have been worse. As I had no retirement savings invested, at least I hadn't taken the kind of hit that most mid- or late-career workers had. I remember Dad telling me that he and Mom had lost nearly half of their retirement savings in the span of a year or so. Already in his fifties and with dreams of retiring while he was still young enough to live a life of continued adventure, travel, and competition, Dad knew he didn't have a lot of years left to make up the shortfall. His answer was to work harder and bill more hours. His 4:30 a.m. alarm was reset to 3:30. Some days were even earlier, and he worked through the night at the office with regularity. Katelyn and I were supporting ourselves by then, but Dona was still at home and my parents wanted to travel during retirement, so Dad felt the pressure to bill, bill, bill. He remained engaged in family and training, but sleep was sacrificed even more than in the past. Just a few years before we started learning about how important sleep is for so many functions, including scrubbing the brain of waste products that may contribute to cognitive decline, Dad's daily schedule had moved sleep deprivation from something experienced occasionally in races to a chronic presence.

One of the best things about living in the Colorado mountains was that I could compete in a wide range of races without having to travel very far. Snowshoe and mountain bike races were often held at nearby ski areas or in the vicinity of outdoor athletic hubs like Leadville or the Vail Valley. I continued to win or finish strong in a good number of the races I entered, particularly snowshoe races. I won the Colorado State Championship four times between 2008 and 2012. (Meanwhile, Dad was still collecting first-place medals in masters' snowshoe races around the state.) A mountain biking highlight for me was setting a new course record while winning the Silver Rush 50-mile mountain bike race in Leadville in 2010.

I also ventured to competitions in neighboring states. In 2009 and again in 2010, I won the Mt. Taylor Quadrathlon, a New Mexico race that includes road biking, running, skiing, and snowshoeing to the summit of 11,306-foot Mt. Taylor and then turning around and doing it all in reverse. When my schedule permitted, I'd squeeze in quick trips to Utah for trail marathons and mountain bike races.

I frequently got the chance to go farther afield to

compete in mountain bike or adventure races in British Columbia, Europe, Brazil, or, memorably in 2009, all the way to the United Arab Emirates to compete in the Abu Dhabi Adventure Challenge, another race descended from the original Raid Gauloises—the event that spawned the entire sport of adventure racing. Our squad, Team Salomon/ Crested Butte, an amalgam of past sponsors and athletes, joined forty teams representing twenty countries in sea kayaking, swimming, biking, and running in the six-day stage race. It's an experience I will never forget, particularly the 60-mile trek across the dunes and salt flats of Abu Dhabi's Rub' al Khali, or "Empty Quarter," the largest expanse of unbroken sand in the world. I served as the team's navigator. Atypical for an adventure race—and due to the real possibility of becoming irrevocably lost in the desert—organizers allowed GPS navigation for this leg of the race. But when our GPS unit's battery died in the middle of the desert, I resorted to old-school map and compass—not easy given the ever-shifting sands and lack of waypoints. In a true sprint to the finish (after almost twenty-four hours for this segment), our team won the stage, something I still count as one of the top moments in my adventure racing career.

Though we always rooted for each other, and crewed for each other as often as we could, Dad and I never had the chance to compete on the same team in an adventure race. It's something I'd always regretted. We did, however, get to race together against each other in 2008 in a memorable race in Canada's Northwest Territory called the Rock and Ice Ultra, a foot/ski/snowshoe stage race (choose your conveyance) across the ice-covered lakes and waterways of Canada's Northwest Territory, beginning on Great Slave Lake, the ninth largest lake in the world. In this, one of the coldest, driest outposts in the world, where wolves and moose far outnumber people, nighttime temperatures reach -50°F, while daytime temps might "warm up" to -15°F.

The race covered 140 miles in six stages over the same number of days. At the end of each stage, racers bedded down in a large communal canvas tent with a snow floor but (critically) a wood-burning stove. Water was provided, but racers carried all other supplies and food on a sled behind them. Mine weighed about forty pounds. Sound fun? Well, it did to me, and to Dad, too. When Mom pointed out that pulling a heavy sled for 140 miles might not be ideal for his chronic back pain (herniated disc) and helpfully, hopefully suggested that he opt instead to compete in the ultra's three-day course (the rough equivalent of back-to-back-to-back marathons), he dismissed the notion out of hand, saying that he didn't want to travel all that way for a "three-day fun run." Hello, tree—apple here!

Perhaps not surprisingly, just a handful of racers opted for the race's expedition-length course. I entered intent on winning, but I also looked forward to spending each night in the big tent with Dad and the other racers. It actually all carried a sense of destiny for me. You see, Amy and I were steadily moving toward marriage by that point, and the race's first-place prize was a one-carat diamond (worth around $13,000, or almost half of my annual teaching salary) from the Ekati Diamond Mine north of Yellowknife. As I trained for the race, I visualized my triumphant homecoming proposal, presenting my beloved with the champion's diamond set in a platinum band. All I had to do was win.

Unfortunately, that fairy-tale scenario ran into something like a sub-Arctic buzz saw in the person of Greg McHale. Greg was not unknown to me; I'd raced against him in numerous international adventure races, and I knew him to be a worthy adversary. What I hadn't quite counted on going into the race was how his resident status—he and his wife, Denise, lived and trained year-round in the Yukon—would work so heavily in his favor. In addition to being a superbly gifted and strong endurance athlete, Greg also had a tweaked-out, lightweight, ski-mounted sled that made my flimsy plastic rig look like I'd snatched it off a runny-nosed kid on the nearest sledding hill. Equipment matters, as does homework and field testing, and Greg had me beat on all fronts. I nipped at his heels every day, but at the end of each stage I found myself a little farther behind. Barring calamity, which you never hope for in such circumstances (especially in conditions like these, which made Moab or Sweden look like the kiddie pool), I was racing for second.

Though the field of competitors began as a ragtag collection of strangers (a French-Canadian pilot, a marine in the British Royal Navy, a firefighter from Edmonton, the McHales, Dad and me, and a few others), spending each post-stage night in the same tent with folks who share a gleeful compulsion to suffer lent the whole endeavor an esprit de corps that keeps many in the ultraendurance community coming back time after time. Though fierce competitors by day, we spent our nights thawing out and amiably swapping tales around the fire. We all had stories to tell, but Dad's invariably got the most laughs, and twelve years later, I can still close my eyes and hear his vivid, joyful accounts of running 150 miles through the Sahara at the Marathon des Sables ("hotter'n crap"); having his toenails removed to solve once and for all the problem of subungual hematoma ("best thing I ever did"); getting thrown off a horse at the starting gun of an Eco-Challenge ("Mark Burnett likes a chaotic start"); or getting hopelessly lost among the hoodoos of Moab ("We were in the wrong damn canyon!"). It never sounded like bragging. It was always self-deprecating, always playful, frequently punctuated with Class B Misdemeanor curse words—just pure, unfiltered Mark Macy. A decade later, when I joined Greg up north to film a couple episodes as a guest on his adventure hunting TV show, *Greg McHale's Wild Yukon*, we spent three weeks out in the woods imitating Dad every time we poked our head into the tent: "Shit, it's cold out there! Man, why didn't anyone tell me my back would hurt so fucking bad?!" Dad finished the Rock and Ice Ultra somewhere in the middle of the small pack (but finished, as usual, herniated disc and all), and me, well, I headed back to Colorado with the second-place prize—no diamond, just a handshake and a pat on the back.

No matter—I still went home and proposed to Amy, and on a gorgeous September day among the changing aspen leaves we were married at the top of a ski lift at Copper Mountain, Colorado. The next year, we bought a house in Evergreen, the hidden-away mountain hamlet where I was raised and my parents still lived. I'd now be training on the same forested mountain trails and roads that had brought Dad so much joy and solitude over the years. And the fact that it was 3,000 feet higher in elevation than Denver could only help my own training and fitness. I also got a job teaching at my alma mater, just down the hall from my old basketball coach, Scott Haebe, and helped out periodically as a volunteer track coach on the team he was coaching in the spring.

The year 2008 ended on a high note for Dad, too (and really for our whole family), when he joined his Stray Dogs team-mate Marshall Ulrich for the final leg of his 3,000-mile run across America. At age fifty-seven, Marshall was attempting to set a new speed record for the transcontinental crossing. While his time of 52.5 days was fast enough to place him third all-time, he did set new masters' and grand masters' speed records. His mind-blowing accomplishment was the equivalent of running two marathons plus a 10k every day for fifty-two straight days. Dad and I joined Marsh for a couple days of running while he made his way across Colorado. Most dramatic, and frankly surreal, was the finish. Dad met up with Marshall in eastern Pennsylvania and would stay with him for the final few days of the run. On the last day, as a documentary film crew followed along, they ran across the Hudson River on the George Washington Bridge into Manhattan. (As Marshall notes in his book, Dad stayed back to let him trot across the bridge alone.) The date, November 4, 2008, is historic for another reason. It was election day—the day Barack Obama won his first term as president. Needless to say, the scene in New York City that late afternoon was a little raucous. Picking their way down Broadway and through Times Square, Marshall and Dad ran right into the heart of the biggest party of the year. "Cars and cabs were gridlocked on the streets with horns blaring," says Dad, "and the cameraman and I were jumping and climbing over parked cars. It was the craziest thing you ever saw."

Marshall's book, subtitled *An Ultramarathoner's Story of Love, Loss, and a Record-Setting Run across America,* does a meticulous job of capturing the toll it takes on a body to accomplish such a feat. And, to his credit, Marshall is unflinchingly honest about the toll his commitment to ultra-running has also taken on his relationships with his wives (two divorces) and children. In one section of the book, he writes of his admiration for my dad. I'll never forget how proud I felt reading it for the first time, and I can attest to its truth 100 percent.

Still, Mace has done a better job with balancing the needs of his family and his own aspirations than I have. I continue to learn from him, including how positive relationships and great athletic achievement can actually complement one another, building courage, confidence, and perseverance for both. Even though he's a couple years younger than I am, he's a mentor to me, showing me how a man can both honor his family and follow his dreams, how he can be emotionally open and still a fierce competitor in the field—a temperance and temperament I have yet to master. His wife and children always come first.

In 2011, I was twenty-eight years old and a five-year veteran high school English teacher. I was still entering as many races (adventure, trail-running, mountain biking, snowshoeing, ski mountaineering) as I could fit into my schedule. But that schedule got a lot more full on January 2 with the arrival of our first child. I was stoked to be a dad and dreamed of sharing all the fun, adventurous, empowering experiences with Wyatt that my dad had shared with me. First-time-parent years are wonder years. (I wonder why he's crying?...I wonder if I'll ever get a full night's sleep again?) Kidding there, kind of. If you're a parent, you know what I mean. Becoming a parent changes you in ways you could never imagine. I remember once seeing a quote that read: "Making the decision to have a child—it is momentous. It is to decide forever to have your heart go walking around outside your body." (I looked it up, and it was written by Elizabeth Stone—a teacher, naturally.) So right. I also learned that parenting was kind of like being married or signing up for an adventure race: you're quite sure you want to do this big thing, but in truth you have absolutely no idea what you're getting into until you start doing it. Getting advice and reading books (parenting continues to be one of my favorite genres) are helpful, but you really have to learn by doing it. And just when you think you have it figured out, your kid gets older (and so do you and your own parents).

Becoming a parent certainly can trigger reflection and soul-searching—especially during those sleep-interrupted nights. My first year as a parent/teacher/ultra-athlete had its rough moments, particularly on the athlete side. With high expectations, my adventure racing team traveled to China to compete in two prominent races but finished a disappointing fourth in both. I tried not to doubt myself and my own contribution to the team. I tried not to envy the freedom of my childless competitors. I tried not to stress about losing corporate sponsorship as an athlete. I tried not to freak out about my impending thirtieth birthday. I tried not to resent the fact that my still-frozen teaching salary was making me feel frustrated and stagnant in my job. But doubt was creeping in.

The one thing beyond doubt was that I loved being a dad. Good thing, too, because our second child, a daughter, was due shortly after Wyatt's second birthday. In my first book, I wrote about this tipping point in my life in the context of the power of the stories we tell ourselves. The story that was creeping in for me bore the depressing headline "The End of Travis Macy's Adventure Career."

But that story was never written. (And I don't intend for it to be for a long time!) By the end of the following year, I had retooled my approach to competing, largely opting for shorter solo races that didn't require traveling to the other side of the globe—or could include Amy and the kids if they did. Even better, I set my own challenge by attempting an FKT, or fastest known time, for running forty-eight miles across the wilderness of Utah's Zion National Park. The FKT phenomenon, facilitated by the broad availability of GPS watches and apps, had recently caught the imagination of the running and biking community, myself included. For me, it was the perfect way to compete "against the world" at a time and under circumstances that best suited my schedule.

The previous FKT for running across Zion, set by elite ultrarunner Luke Nelson, was 7 hours, 48 minutes. On the morning of April 6, 2013, with no cheering crowds and a spartan crew of two—my neighbor Charles Martelli (whom I had recently begun coaching for his first ultra) and his brother-in-law Nick Yaskoff—I pushed a button on my watch and set off from the west edge of the park. What lay ahead was a linked patchwork of trails over sand, rock, mud, slickrock, and riverbed with climbs and descents that would total 10,000 vertical feet.

My run across the park was not exactly a walk in the park, but all in all I enjoyed pushing my body to the limit on a beautiful spring day in such a breathtaking place. I also rather enjoyed the fleeting, dumbfounded looks from tourists as I blew past them in the park's more populated areas. As the morning cold gave way to afternoon heat and fresh legs became heavy, I talked to myself: "Hang tough, Trav. The farther we go, the stronger we get. It's all good mental training, Trav. Keep the faith." Sometimes the inner voice was mine; sometimes it sounded like Dad. As the clock ticked down in my last few miles of running, I felt good about my chances of besting Luke's FKT, but nothing was assured. As I wrote in *The Ultra Mindset:*

I considered my stories. One of the narratives involved me staggering to a halt, cramped up or bonking; taken down by a course too long, hilly, and hot for a thirty-year-old high-school teacher and father of two kids in diapers. The other narrative grew louder with each step: this was essentially the story I'm telling you now, about how I had set this goal as a way to launch a new direction in my life as an endurance athlete. It was me, in the wilderness I loved, alone and racing against the clock.

When I crossed the finish line—which wasn't an actual finish line but instead the eastern boundary of the national park marked by an old rusty gate—I pushed the button on my watch: 7 hours, 27 minutes. I had broken the Zion traverse record by over twenty minutes. But more importantly, I had emerged from a figurative wilderness as well as a literal one. My time would be broken a few weeks later, but I didn't care: My new story had begun.

The next chapter of that story would be an ultraendurance challenge I had dreamed about for years. The setting, not surprisingly given my family history, was Leadville, Colorado: altitude 10,151 feet; population 2,600 and change.

Leadville. That word had first entered my consciousness when I was five years old. More than just a town on a map, Leadville loomed as an emotional and psychological destination, just as the aptly and unambiguously named Mount Massive looms over the town itself. Leadville was the place where a shotgun blast had jarred me from bleariness at 4:00 a.m. in 1988, standing in the middle of the street in my footed jammies, snow boots, and winter jacket, watching with a mix of confusion and absolute absorption as hundreds of lean adults stared down headlamp beams into darkness, bounced on their toes, jogged in place for warmth, and then, at the shot, set off, swallowed up by that predawn darkness. My dad had been among them that year. By the time I watched him hobble back into town nearly thirty hours later, a bearing had been set on my own psychological compass.

By 2013, I had already competed in plenty of races in and around Leadville—trail running, snowshoeing, mountain biking—but I hadn't committed to the granddaddy of them all: the Leadville 100 Trail Run, the "Race Across the Sky." By then, this race had become a family legacy. Dad had run it five times between 1988 and 1995, but that was just the Macy side. Beginning in the early '90s, my mom's side of the family had racked up around twenty-five finishes, led by my uncle Eric, who had his eighteenth finish in 2012. He's still running, by the way. He notched his twenty-sixth finish in the summer of 2021. My uncle Brian, who donated a kidney to my mom in 2002, had finished; and Eric's wife, Anne, and Mom's brother-in-law, Tim, have also finished the race. Eric's son, my cousin Ethan, has also since joined the group, getting his first finish in 2018.

Growing up around all this, it was clearly just a matter of time before I got in on the type II fun, and in some ways I'm surprised it had taken me until 2013 to commit to the race. Part of the reason I waited was because I wanted to do more than just the 100-miler (and, yes, I realize how ridiculous that sounds. As they used to say on late-night infomercials, "But wait!... There's more!"). Welcome, folks, to the ADD/adventure/competition/perfectionism mind. I am thankful to say I've learned a lot about the good and bad components of my wiring and conditioning, such that doing less and gaining wisdom are now often more important than doing more and notching results.

Oh boy, though, was there more! Twenty years after the Leadville Trail 100's debut in 1983, the race's cofounder, Ken Chlouber, came up with the idea of expanding the single race into a series of five races that would span six weeks of the summer. The lineup of races is as follows. Each race is contested at elevations between 10,200 and 13,186 feet.

1. trail-running marathon (26.2 miles)
2. (two weeks later) 50-mile mountain bike race or 50-mile trail run
3. (a little less than a month later) 100-mile mountain bike race
4. (the day after that) 10k road race
5. (the next weekend) the Leadville 100 trail run

Any athlete who successfully finishes each race in the series (beating the cutoff time for each) earns the title Leadman or Leadwoman. In 2013, I set my sights on not only earning that title but winning the Leadman competition by compiling the fastest cumulative time across the five events. Hey, if you're gonna go, you might as well go big.

Sometimes people assume Dad pushed me toward endurance racing in general and Leadville in particular. That's not the case; I loved the experience and achievement, and the drive came from within. Nonetheless, Mom and Dad were definitely part of my Leadman team. Dad and Uncle Eric provided valuable input on mindset and strategy. Yeah, I was a well-established athlete and coach, but these guys had done the Leadville 100 Run—and I hadn't. Mom, Amy, and Sandy (Amy's mom) chipped in for extra support and flexibility with childcare so I could train more.

The series started off well. I battled a strong field in the marathon. (Silly to say, really. Every race in the series had a strong field as athletes come from across the globe to compete in Leadville—and the large-lunged locals are often even better than the international pros.) I kept to my pacing and hydration/nutrition strategy and finished in second place, less than two minutes behind the winner, Marshall Thomson, who had also won the marathon the previous year. If you're a road runner and my time of 3:38:52 sounds slow, come on up to the big hill in the thin air next year to see how fast you can "run."

The Silver Rush 50 mountain bike race two weeks later wasn't my best outing. Three years earlier I had won this race while setting a course record, but this time, after leading early, I found myself passed by a long line of riders who had conserved energy by working together and drafting off me—a tried and true cycling strategy. I recovered strength and position later in the race and managed a ninth-place finish—good enough to keep me in the top spot among the Leadman racers.

Four weeks later, I was back in Leadville and back on the bike for the 100-miler. I needed all the positive stories and voices in my head I could get during this grueling race. During big climbs—which is where I'm usually at my best in mountain bike races—I'd repeat a mantra to myself:

The higher we go, the stronger we get. Come on, Trav.

As the course reached past 75, 80, 90 miles and I pushed to maintain position at the front of the Leadman field, I tweaked it slightly:

The longer we go, the stronger we get. Come on, Trav.

I had more than just the voices in my head in this race. I had Dad, who was crewing for me. Just as valuable as the fresh bottles he'd hand me at feed zones were his words of encouragement, lifted straight off the script from our climbs up the hills behind our house when I was a little kid: "It's all good mental training, Bud. Overcome the fear, Bud. Commit to it. Crush those hills! The higher you go, the stronger you get." Yup, so many of those voices that kept me going traced straight back to Dad.

I kept replaying that track and kept pushing all the way back to town, and as I cranked up 6th Street toward the finish—first among the Leadman contenders (our race bibs identified us with a big black L), the crowd on the street went crazy. At 7 hours, 32 minutes, I was 23 minutes ahead of the second Leadman racer and still holding on to the overall lead with three races down and two to go.

Dad and I camped out together that weekend, as usual, in my funky old travel trailer. No heat or appliances, but it kept out most of the rain and gave us a spot to hang out together. He navigated the crowds on the bike course to hand me bottles at miles 40 and 60, and after the race we drove together to Copper Mountain so I could deliver a clinic on adventure racing for the athletes who were competing in a local series. Crew for you all day in a 100-mile bike race and then go to an evening clinic to support you there? That might have been a lot to ask of most sixty-year-old fathers, but Dad didn't question it or miss a beat.

The fourth race in the series—the 10k run—would be almost a lark, if it weren't held the day after a 100-mile bike race and a week before the 100-mile trail run. My strategy was to take it easy and give up a few minutes in overall time in exchange for conserving my strength for the LT100 and avoiding injury. First, of course, I had to drag myself out of bed the day after racing a hundred miles on the bike. Fortunately, motivation to do so was not lacking. I let the leaders go hard and enjoyed a pretty leisurely pace, keeping my powder dry for the following weekend.

I'd love to say I spent the week leading up to the Leadville 100 run perfecting an innovative recovery strategy to be shared with my coaching clients, but I didn't—because I was at work as a high school teacher. I recall a couple of phone calls. In one of them, my friend Dave Mackey, an accomplished ultrarunner, advised wisely: "Trav, if you think you might be going out too fast, then you are. Just take it easy and be patient." Good advice. And in the other call, Mom and Dad said pretty much the usual things: "We love you and we're proud of you no matter what. Just do your best, and we're excited to be in Leadville with you."

When I first imagined myself as a Leadman competitor several years before, I knew the 100-mile run would be the key. An athlete can melt down in the 100 bike and lose an hour; falling apart in the run could easily slow a racer by five hours or more. This was the one that would test my body. I'd never run a hundred miles before. This was the one that would test my spirit. Running nonstop, alone, at elevations in excess of 12,000 feet, what voices would I hear? What story would they tell me? This was the one that would test my will. Would I have the grit not to give up when my body and mind were both begging me to do just that?

On August 18, 2013, whether triumphant or heartbroken, I was bound to write the next chapter in my story. Twenty-five years earlier I'd stood on this same corner of 6th and Harrison in the predawn hours waiting anxiously and sleepily for my dad to start this race—part of a much smaller field. No jammies this time, and I wasn't sleepy. I was amped up. I'd awoken that morning in my junky, old, cold travel trailer and read Dr. Seuss's *Oh, the Places You'll Go!* to myself. Out loud. When Ken Chlouber's shotgun fired, I was off with the pack. Here we go! Off to great places…I hope. Be back in a hundred miles.

My plan was to start conservatively and not get caught up in racing early on. Station to station, mile by mile, I'd break the run down into manageable chunks and maintain my pace. About a quarter of the way in, I was somewhere in the thirties in the field of around 1,000 runners. Approaching the middle of the race, up and over the high point of Hope Pass, I passed more runners, feeling strong. I was happy to see my family at the ghost town of Winfield (but passed on the family picnic we'd had with Dad twenty-five years earlier). Near Winfield, the course reversed and we headed back toward Leadville, still nearly fifty miles away.

Shortly thereafter, things started to get shaky. My top two rivals for the Leadman crown, my friends Bob Africa and Luke Jay, passed me on the way back down Hope Pass. I caught them again on the next climb, and we were running as a pack at the 60-mile mark. I listened to their breathing and stole an occasional glance. Bob and Luke were both sounding strong and moving well, but I was starting to suffer. I had become slightly dehydrated in the afternoon heat and nausea soon followed. I'd never run this far in my life, and now...well, I was barely running at all. The voices in my head were not helping. After seventy miles of running, I was teetering on the brink of physical and emotional meltdown.

As I plodded on, I thought about how I would explain my situation to Dad at the next aid station. How my legs were trashed and I was dehydrated. How every step hurt. How my main Leadman rival, Bob Africa, blew past me miles ago, looking as strong and comfortable as he did at the start.

I knew this was the crux of the race, but I felt that it was even more—the defining moment of my own story. My story, inextricably linked with Dad's story, Mom's story, Amy's story, the story I'd tell my children and they might tell theirs someday.

I shuffled on. A new voice whispered, a voice I knew well.

Don't quit.

The nugget of all Dad's axioms boiled down to two words. Another voice.

You're better than you think you are. You can do more than you think you can.

Ken Chlouber's traditional prerace pep talk.

But am I? Can I?

Don't quit.

It became my new mantra. I kept running.

Don't quit.

I kept running, and I started to feel stronger.

Don't quit.

The sun set. The day cooled, and, with it, the tumult in my mind.

Don't quit.

Months ago, years ago, I had committed to this and told myself that quitting was not an option.

Though still twenty-five miles from Leadville, I conjured a finish line in my mind. But it wasn't the finish line of this race. It was the finish line of Dad's first Leadville 100, twenty-five years ago. I saw him shuffling up 6th Street on his own trashed legs. At five years old, I hadn't known how much he was suffering. Now I knew. Dad was finishing last, but he was finishing with a spirit undaunted. *Don't quit.* And I wouldn't. I would find my own finish line.

I also remembered I wasn't alone. Mom, Dad, Amy, Katelyn, Dona, Sandy, and Steve; my coach, Josiah Middaugh; my friends and pacers—they were all in this with me, too. We were a team. Adventure racing teammate and close friend Shane Sigle was pacing me now, and he knew just what to do

"Trav, eat this Cheeto."

He waited for no response before reaching across and

literally shoving the orange, salty, crunchy, food-like item in my mouth. I grunted but didn't puke, so he kept doing that every couple of minutes until I actually had some energy again.

A few hours later, I pushed across the line with tears in my eyes and my heart full of joy. My time of 20 hours, 15 minutes was good enough for fifteenth place in the run. Over the course of the six-week Leadville Race Series I had run and biked 282.4 miles and climbed 44,951 feet in 36 hours and 20 minutes. I had won the series and set a new record. I hadn't quit. I had won. I was a Leadman.

In the wake of my Leadman victory, my life changed and it didn't change. I achieved a brief level of acclaim and notoriety (at least in the world of endurance sports) that I had never experienced before. Media interviews, new sponsorship opportunities, new coaching clients (including a few fellow Leadmen, like Bob, whom I coached to the win the next year) who wanted my guidance in helping them achieve their own ultrarunning and endurance goals. But it wasn't like I won the Super Bowl. There was no fat paycheck or new long-term contract waiting to be signed. I collected my LT100 belt buckle. Someone mailed me a neat bumper sticker for my truck, reading Pb Man, which is surely meaningless to 99.9 percent of people who see it—other than residents of Park County, Colorado. (But I never get tired of seeing it!) I went home to Evergreen with my wife and two kids. I kept running, kept biking, and started to think about what was next.

Shortly thereafter, Amy and I both shifted from traditional employment with schools to self-employment, with her building the independent postsecondary transition counseling business she still runs today, and me focusing on coaching adult endurance athletes, speaking, writing, and racing. We enjoyed a six-week trip to Europe in the summer of 2014. Wyatt was three and Lila one; Amy's mom, Sandy, joined to help with the kids and feed her own love of travel. The time with our friends from adventure racing, Emma and David, in the Catalonian Pyrenees was incredible. I got to compete in some neat trail running races in France, including the Vertical Kilometer World Championship (straight uphill, gaining 1,000 vertical meters in less than 40 minutes), where I finished seventh. That was a special race for me because Mom, Dad, Katelyn, and Dona had flown to Chamonix to support me, and everyone ascended the ski hill in a gondola that traveled above me. I could hear them cheering and pounding on the gondola as they passed above, and they were waiting at the finish when I arrived. Pretty cool! In hindsight, that moment of peaceful triumph looks like a calm before a storm that would include health challenges, diagnoses, and a concussion that increased my anxiety and depression. Lessons learned: be present; enjoy what you have; don't take it for granted; invest in building a team that can support each other when things get tough.

Over the following few years, I focused on ultra-running as a sponsored HOKA ONE ONE athlete, competing in events like the HURT 100 in Hawaii, the Wasatch 100 in Utah, and the San Juan Solstice 50 in Colorado, among others. Mom and Dad crewed many of those, and I had a blast with Amy's dad, Steve, as he crewed all night long in Hawaii. Some people complain about their in-laws, but mine are the best! They continue to play a big role in supporting me, Dad, Mom, and Amy in the Alzheimer's journey.

Amy and I often joke about how different our families were growing up. Her parents were hyperorganized—again, the apple/tree axiom holds true. Before a family vacation, they would outline every detail, plan a route, book rooms, schedule each day's activities.... My parents, well, they weren't overplanners, or even really planners. When Friday came, we'd all jump in the car and off we'd go. When one of us kids would ask where we were going, the answer was, as often as not, "We'll know when we get there."

Mom and Dad have always been adventurous, so when Dad told us in 2015 that he was going to retire from his law firm at the end of the year, and that he and Mom were going to buy a travel trailer and hit the road, I wasn't at all surprised. Dad had been a successful attorney for more than thirty years, but anyone who knew him well knew that his identity wasn't wrapped up in the career. Lawyering was a job for Dad, and he had no trouble with the notion of walking away. In fact, he had been excited to do so for years! There was just so much to do—so many back roads to explore and trails to run. My sister Dona had graduated high school a few years earlier and moved out of the house in Evergreen, so Mom and Dad were free and clear to get out and explore. I was thrilled for them.

I didn't know it at the time, but Mom would tell me later that Dad's decision to retire may have been reinforced by a nascent insecurity about his job performance. Beginning in 2015, he started to notice that in depositions he would—not always, but occasionally—lose his train of thought and have to mentally press a reset on a line of questioning. Any worries Dad might have had he kept largely to himself. The only one he would confide in was Mom. "He couldn't explain why," she says, "he just didn't feel like he was on top of his game." Dad's concern was great enough that he agreed to get an MRI in late 2015. "It came back completely normal," Mom recalls. "The neurologist said, 'There's nothing wrong with you and nothing to worry about.' Neither of us had been particularly worried, but we were relieved just the same. We moved on and didn't think much more about it."

At age sixty-two, Dad wasn't entering as many races—he'd often grumble that there weren't as many snowshoe races as there used to be, which I think might have been a corollary effect of the surging popularity of ski mountaineering—but he was, of course, still running, biking, swimming, and snowshoeing for fun and fitness, and was generally the same paragon of health he had always been.

Still, in the months leading up to and immediately following Dad's retirement, Mom noticed some unsettling things. Because he was a partner in his law firm and because they needed to continue on the firm's health insurance plan, his retirement plan was somewhat complicated. Mom had never gotten involved in the employee benefits side of Dad's job before, but as the two of them were finalizing how the retirement plan would be structured, she noticed that Dad was unable to hold on to the details. Here was the guy who, for decades, had been negotiating minutiae like insurance benefits on behalf of his entire firm. "We made jokes about it," Mom recalls, "like, boy, you got out of there just in time, but it was startling. It was the first time I thought maybe there really was something going on."

A few months later, on one of their first trips in the new trailer, she caught another glimpse of what would become their new reality. "We were at a rest area looking at the map," Mom recalls, "and he couldn't read the map... and that was, to me... I was almost, like, gasping, because he's always had this incredible internal navigation system no matter where we were. In Europe... before the days of cell phones and GPS navigation... he was just really good at that. So the fact that he couldn't read this map—couldn't tell what was north, south, east, and west—that was just another moment of realization." Still, Mom didn't make too much of that or similar instances. "I wanted him to come to the conclusion that we should look into testing, not me," she says.

Even as Mom worried about Dad's lapses in clarity and memory, she was also dealing with her own health problems. It had been nearly fifteen years since she had received a kidney donation from her brother, Uncle Brian. A living, related, donor kidney (the best possible kind) functions on average from twelve to twenty years.

Mom got lab work done every six weeks, as is typical for donor kidney recipients, and the trend line wasn't good. Still, as her condition slowly deteriorated, she never complained. That had never been her way. "You can feel okay even though you're not at your best," she explains. "You can manage and still get through the day."

That kind of compartmentalizing works up to a point, just as it did with Dad's cognitive slips, but in the summer of 2017 Mom's health reached a tipping point. While on a Mediterranean cruise, Mom contracted a virus of some kind and got alarmingly ill. By the time they reached port, she was highly anemic, weak, and chronically short of breath. Back home, her nephrologist immediately admitted Mom to the hospital. Her kidney function was around 20 percent, the range that qualifies for a transplant.

Dad's blood type is incompatible with Mom's, making him ineligible to donate one of his own kidneys, but several months earlier they had researched the possibility of entering the paired exchange program through the National Kidney Registry and the University of Colorado Anschutz Medical Campus in Denver. Such programs involve two living donors and two recipients, as explained on the National Kidney Foundation's website:

If the recipient from one pair is compatible with the donor from the other pair, and vice versa—the transplant center may arrange for a "swap"—for two simultaneous transplants to take place. This allows two transplant candidates to receive organs and two donors to give organs though the original recipient/donor pairs were unable to do so with each other.

After undergoing extensive physical testing, Dad was accepted into the nationwide paired donor system. That's not easy to do. Only one out of every eight applicants ends up qualifying. But despite being sixty-four years old (in 2017), Dad's physical fitness meant that his kidney was worthy to pass along to someone in need. His willingness to donate to a stranger meant that Mom would A) receive an organ from a living donor rather than a cadaver, and B) likely have a shorter wait to receive that organ.

But by the summer of 2017, Mom could no longer wait to be matched up within the paired donor system. Her kidney was failing, and if functionality dipped to 10 percent she'd need to begin dialysis, something she and all of us desperately wanted to avoid. Dad looked to my uncle Eric, mom's youngest brother, for help. Uncle E has always had a nonchalant approach toward endeavors like running a hundred miles in the mountains, and it turned out he reacted similarly to the idea of getting an organ taken out of his body. After finishing a snowshoe race in Leadville:

"Eric, what do you think about donating a kidney to Pammy?"

Two seconds of consideration.

"Sure, Mace, I'll do that."

That was that, and testing a few days later showed he was a match.

In December of 2017, Eric and Mom underwent transplant surgery, and it was another happy nonending for the Macy/Pence clan. Just as she had after receiving her first donated kidney, Mom immediately felt more robust. I'll never forget Mom's pale visage going into surgery; and then the anxious hours waiting in the hospital during the transplant; and finally the relief when, incredibly, her face again showed a vibrant and natural color even as the anesthesia wore off. Organ transplants are incredible (and I highly encourage you to declare donation eligibility on your driver's license if you have not). As for my Uncle Eric, he felt good enough that just eight months after donating his kidney and saving Mom's life, he went out and finished yet another Leadville 100 trail race. Mom loves to say that for a few years she had the most Leadville finishes in the family, if you counted the contribution of all of her donated parts, because when Uncle Brian donated kidney #1, he had finished the race four times and when Uncle Eric donated #2, he had done it twenty-three times. So, Mom's kidneys had run the 100-miler twenty-seven times!

Because Mom ultimately received a kidney from outside the paired donor program, Dad was off the hook, no longer obligated to donate one of his. I don't know if my dad believes in karma, but I do know, with 100 percent certainty, that he believes in doing the right thing. Six months after Mom received her kidney, Dad checked into University of Colorado Anschutz Medical Campus and donated one of his kidneys to a fifty-one-year-old Kansas farmer with hereditary polycystic kidney disease—a disease that had killed the man's own father. As it turns out, the recipient was a fan of the Eco-Challenge race series and was thrilled to learn that he would be receiving such a badass replacement organ. Mom and Dad remain in close contact with the recipient, who to this day calls his donor kidney "Little Mace."

Talk of kidney function and kidney donation had dominated the conversation within my family in 2017 and the first half of 2018, but a different anxiety, left largely unexpressed, still lurked beneath the surface. Quietly, Mom had approached my sisters and me about Dad's mental state, asking if we had noticed any changes. We all had our own stories to add to Mom's litany of concerns. Sometimes it was trouble with word finding, or he'd be unable to come up with a long-familiar name. At other times I noticed less certainty in his navigation when driving and inconsistencies in his speed on the highway. Dad typically played off such momentary lapses, dismissing them as "just typical old-guy stuff" (as if Dad was ever a typical old guy), but it was obviously frustrating and worrisome to him.

Dad is one of the most positive people I've ever known— not in a Pollyannaish way but just in a "things will work out if you work hard and don't let yourself get down" kind of way. Still, I imagine that, like most of us, he sometimes let his mind slip toward those darker places and wondered if his mental lapses were born of a more sinister source. And what if he did have some kind of cognitive impairment? He was old enough to have known plenty of people whose lives had been touched by Alzheimer's and other forms of dementia. He knew the stark reality. No treatment, no cure. So, what the hell's the rush in finding out bad news? And Dad had a secondary reason for putting off testing. He was determined to wait until after he had donated a kidney before seeking answers from the medical profession. He wanted to repay the selflessness of donors who had come to Mom's rescue three times in the past. He wanted to pay it forward. And he knew it was unlikely the transplant team would allow him to do so if he were diagnosed with some kind of cognitive disorder.

Dad's sister, Aunt Boo, recalls family gatherings from around that time, noticing her brother go quiet and withdraw when conversations got crowded and raucous. Normally, he would have been right in the thick of things, telling stories and cracking jokes. "You could see it in his eyes," she says. "It was like he was afraid he couldn't finish a sentence if he tried to converse."

Dad and Mom finally went to a neurologist for testing in October of 2018. By this time, I had already nearly worn out my laptop's search engine trying to learn all I could about dementia in general and Alzheimer's specifically. I had read books by experts and research papers published in medical journals. None of it made me feel better. The more I learned, the more Dad's aberrant behavior made sense. But until there was a diagnosis, I still held out hope. That's why I didn't blame Dad for delaying a diagnosis. You could think something all day long and assume the worst, but until you heard a definitive statement from a medical expert, you could still hold on to that hope. (For what it's worth, I have since learned that early identification greatly expands treatment options and potential for mild cognitive impairment, Alzheimer's, and other dementias. So, if you're reading this and think you or someone you care about might benefit from testing, please, PLEASE, initiate the tough conversations and take action. NOW. Not later.)

On October 16, 2018, with a call from my mom on the way home from Dad's appointment, any hope that the symptoms might not mean anything was snuffed out. People of my grandfather's generation knew exactly where they were when they learned of Pearl Harbor. For my generation, it was the attack on the Twin Towers. But for some reason I don't remember the precise moment my mom called. I know, though, that I wasn't surprised. Not surprised, but still destroyed. Is it possible to not be surprised but still be shocked? That's what I felt in the wake of the call. Shock. Shock that such a world-exploding diagnosis could be rendered so swiftly and definitively. Shock that the man who had always shown me the way, who had always helped me find the answers, would no longer be able to find his own way, and that there were no answers. No treatment, no cure, no answers. No course of action. This is perhaps what I felt most keenly of all in that moment. I didn't know what the hell to do. Dad and I always considered ourselves men of action. Get out there and do something! Move! Push! Persist! Run farther! Climb higher! Live! How does he live with this, though? How do I?

Once the initial shock (or at least the initial wave of shock) receded, my mind began jumping to future hypotheticals. I felt like I needed to immediately figure out everything financial—to look into power of attorney and make sure Mom's name was on all their accounts. I was desperate to investigate any possible treatment options. Open to anything. I had read *The End of Alzheimer's* by Dale Bredesen (subtitle: *The First Protocol to Enhance Cognition and Reverse Decline at Any Age*), and even though I was skeptical about the strength of the scientific and clinical evidence that guided the protocol, I thought, We gotta get on that full speed, immediately! In hindsight, it feels like I was engaged in a lot of scrambling to try to control the uncontrollable or deny reality.

A few days after the diagnosis, Amy and the kids and I went to Mom and Dad's for a Sunday dinner. I was still reeling. All of us were. We tried to keep the conversation positive, but the darkness loomed around every corner and filled all the empty spaces. We didn't yet talk about Alzheimer's with the kids around. Looking back, I appreciate my parents'

matter-of-fact tone in discussing scary things like liver transplants back in the day. I sought the same tone in discussing
Alzheimer's with Wyatt (then seven) and Lila (then five), but
I wouldn't be capable of using the word "Alzheimer's" with
my kids without completely breaking down for another six
months. Meanwhile, Mom had told me that Dad (with her
help transcribing) had begun keeping a journal to document
his Alzheimer's journey. It didn't surprise me to hear that.
After all, he had always provided detailed postrace wrap-ups
of his most prominent races (like all the Eco-Challenges) to
his sponsors. I was happy to hear he was doing that even if I
was pissed off at the reason. My emotions were just swirling.
Pride, anger, love, helplessness. It scared me to think what
Dad might be writing because I knew that his emotions were
just as raw and mercurial as my own. I hoped he was finding
some solace in his journaling, but I also knew that it would
be a long time (three years, as it turned out) before I was
ready to read what he was putting on the page. Some entries,
like this one, I just couldn't help but smile about:

*At 10 pm last night I opened my iPad and was
surprised to find an email from one of my in-laws.
And was even more surprised at the content of the
email which suggested that due to my recent
diagnosis of Alzheimer's, that I videotape
conversations with my children in which I will save
for posterity the highlights of my life. Her
assumption was that because I have ALZ I would
die soon.*

*My first thought when I read this was "Bullshit!"
and I had no intention of dying and had plenty of
time to tell my stories. This person was only motivated
out of kindness and concern for family.*

Travis and Mark Macy

This family member has been in the medical profession her entire life and has the perspective that there is no effective treatment and that my fate is death. I am not choosing to make a video now. I might get around to it in another twenty years.

When dinner ended, I made some excuse to leave the room—to go warm up the car or something. I needed to breathe in the cool October air. I walked downstairs and out through the garage toward the driveway. Moving slowly, I glanced to my left and stopped in midstride. My eyes moved across the cluttered workbench running the length of the wall. A few errant hand tools: a rubber mallet, a hacksaw, an open box of deck screws, a four-foot level, a stack of leftover ceramic tile, a roll of duct tape—the detritus of an everyday life. But a closer look revealed more than just typical workbench stuff. Overflowing from tubs were helmets, pumps, climbing rope, ice-climbing crampons, backpacks, tents, skis, cycling shoes, and gloves. And as I widened my gaze to take in the wall behind the workbench, I saw more of my dad's real life. He was no handyman. Never has been. The wall was a patchwork of pinned-up race bibs, patches, and paraphernalia. This was no trophy wall with carefully curated mementos meant to impress visitors or feed his own ego. This was the garage, where Dad unpacked his gear after returning from races, stowing equipment in Rubbermaid tubs and haphazardly pinning bibs to the sheetrock wall that has remained unfinished and unpainted since this house was built when I was ten years old.

The race bibs read like a scattershot athletic resume: MARATHON DES SABLES MOROCCO #284... SILVER RUSH 50 MTB #589... '97 IDITASPORT ALASKA—A 100 MILE WILDERNESS RACE #3... LEADVILLE

TRAIL 100 #992... ECO-CHALLENGE FIJI 2002 #74... RACING THE PLANET NEPAL 2011 #124. Another RACING THE PLANET bib, this one from 2007 (GOBI DESERT), unceremoniously pinned with a handful of other numbered bibs under an ice ax. A PRIMAL QUEST bib similarly obscured by a cluster of medals hanging from a nail. One of the medallions is stamped SPARTAN RACE WORLD CHAMPIONSHIPS. Dad always laughed about that one, pointing out that he was the only one in his sixty-plus age group who showed up. I keep scanning the wall, my eyes edged with tears now. More ECO-CHALLENGE patches, a few bibs identified only by a sponsor's logo—Coors, Gatorade, Subaru—and then my eyes freeze on a white bib with the stark black number 413 hanging diagonally, fixed to the wall by a yellow pushpin. DIAMOND ULTRA, the race that Dad and I had done together in Canada's Northwest Territory in 2008. Five days of racing, freezing, laughing around a fire at night—it was the longest race we'd ever done together. "One of the best races I ever went to," I'd heard Dad once tell a friend, "because I got to be with Trav." I closed my eyes and let the tears come. Would there ever be another?

"Fuck, fuck, *fuck*!'"

I'm screaming and smashing a snow shovel against a tree in my front yard. It's a Ponderosa pine, eighteen inches in diameter, at least a hundred years old. It's not impressed.

I drank too much beer (for me, that's three), by myself, in the garage. Then I wandered in the dark woods for an hour, crying the whole time, eyelids swollen and rashed from rubbing in frozen tears. It's winter 2018, just a couple of months since the diagnosis, and I'm low, lost, and alone. The uncertainty is crippling and my mind wallows in worst-case scenarios. Right now, it's more than I can take.

How can I go on without my light and my rock? I know the cycle of life means that at some point parents age and the adult children take care of them—but this is happening way sooner than I thought. I'm not ready to take the lead.

Why did this crisis come so soon? To a guy who works hard, gives generously, and treats people right? I mean, a few months ago, he donated a kidney to a stranger. Saving someone's life by giving part of your body: now that's the quintessential "good guy." This is bullshit, as my dad says in his journal, and it's not fair.

FOUR

When did you know and how did you know it?
When I tell people of my ALZ, they often
ask, when did you know and how did you know
it? Just like everybody else, I started to have
some memory and word-finding problems, which
as I understand it, those symptoms alone don't
necessarily mean you have ALZ, and in fact
those symptoms can be normal. But in my case,
I was a trial lawyer and had to talk to people
every single day and ultimately I started to forget
names and topics of conversation. I was aware I
wasn't the same, but no one else noticed. In fact,
for many people, that may still be the case.
I was well aware of the fact I had cognitive
troubles as early as age sixty, which was two years
before I retired and even mentioned it to a partner,
and the response was always, "There's nothing
wrong with you."

—*MACE'S JOURNAL*

THE EVERGREEN REC CENTER is kind of a second home to Dad. Though he'd always prefer to be training outside, running trails or hammering his mountain bike up one of the dirt roads that spiderweb through the surrounding mountains, he is a regular at the Rec Center too, whether swimming laps, taking yoga classes or a sauna, or just chatting with someone—friend or stranger—who wants to BS for a while.

So when Dad agreed to give a talk on Alzheimer's at the Rec Center in November 2018, he was on his home turf. Mom and I sat up front as Dad stood (or paced, more accurately) before a seated crowd of attendees packed together in a workout room with equipment pushed against the walls.

There were some familiar faces, including Pam Warren, a longtime family friend. She and my mom have hiked together for years in Evergreen, and her daughter Laura and I were student body copresidents our senior year at Evergreen High School. My wife, Amy, sat by Aunt Boo. Marshall Ulrich sat in the back, showing up, as always, to support his old friend, running partner, and teammate, alongside Heather, his wife.

Also in attendance was Peggy Ballengee, a big supporter of mine when I got into adventure racing twenty years ago. I had raced internationally with her daughter, Danelle "Nellie" Ballengee, a world-class multisport athlete who had also grown up in Evergreen. I knew Peggy knew what it was like to face adversity in the family; she had sat beside Nellie's hospital bed in 2006 as she recovered from a near-death fall from a cliff in Moab, Utah, that left her with a shattered pelvis and internal bleeding.

As a teacher, you become adept at reading faces. Looking out at the audience, I noted a range of expressions from curiosity to concern to unmistakable apprehension. No passivity here. These folks were here to learn. Many of them, I surmised, had been touched by Alzheimer's or other forms of dementia or cognitive decline. I may not have known their faces, but I knew their expressions all too well.

In Dad, they were about to hear an honest, endearing, compassionate messenger. Just a little more than a month earlier, he had been on the receiving end of the worst possible news about his cognitive health, delivered in a clinical, matter-of-fact way that had initially left him stunned. He had processed that news, boiled it down to its immutable truths, and then begun to enact his personal response to his condition. In the time since he was diagnosed, Dad had cycled through most, if not all, of the classic steps in the grieving process: denial, anger, depression, acceptance... well, he was still working on acceptance. And I'm pretty sure he skipped bargaining altogether. Now he was ready to share some of what he had experienced.

Dad agreed to do this talk because he maintained something that the medical establishment had not given him much of: hope. He had, just a month before, experienced a feeling that was novel for him, novel in his entire sixty-five years: vulnerability. He'd been given an expiration date, more or less, on his livelihood and his life. Dad, who had dragged himself across the finish line in a 155-mile race through the Sahara Desert, who had discovered unplumbed depths of stamina and will to finish (and win) the 100-mile Iditashoe—snowshoeing in the Alaskan winter—multiple times, did not really accept the word "quit."

Dad quieted the chatter in the room. "You ready?" he said without raising his voice. "You guys ready to go?" The din ceased almost immediately and Dad began his talk. It took him a few minutes to find his rhythm. It had been a handful of years now since he last worked a courtroom as a trial lawyer.

His speech may have been halting at first, a few false starts and a disclaimer about his frequent difficulty with word finding, but his presence captured the audience from the beginning. He looked every bit the world-class athlete that the flyer printed by the Rec Center had promised. Tall. Lean. Ramrod straight through his torso. His quarter-zip black poly-pro shirt bore patches from the Racing the Planet ultra-marathon (250km across the world's most desolate deserts) along with his participant number. His cropped white hair had ceded nothing to the decades. (It had turned white while he was still in his thirties.) A complementary shock of white hair—a "soul patch"—adorned his lower lip. His blue eyes maintained the clarity of youth. He moved with ease in front of the room, amiable and relaxed, never losing eye contact. No notes. No bullshit. I loved seeing him up there even if I hated the reason.

"My name is Mark Macy, and I have early-onset Alzheimer's," he began. "I've been an ultradistance athlete all my adult life. I've run and biked in jungles and deserts. I've kayaked, climbed, and competed all over the world, and I intend to continue on with that. And I believe that I can. I don't think I have to stop because of my Alzheimer's, and I don't intend to. There's just too many things to do in life, and I don't want this disease to stop me or my family or change anything."

Dad didn't try to hide his emotions. Tears would occasionally well in his eyes as he spoke, as if spontaneously triggered by a certain combination of words. Over the preceding months, I had come to know this phenomenon well myself. Neither Dad nor I can stop the sneaker waves of emotion, though each of us can, in most cases, quickly recover our composure.

Dad told the assembled crowd the story of his initial diagnosis, and as he fell into this story, the laughter began.

"The first person that I went to see was recommended to me by a friend. She had a big clock in her office, and she wanted me to draw the clock.

"I thought, '*What the hell?* This is nuts. Anyone can draw a clock.' So I started drawing it, and I finished, and apparently I misplaced the 1 and the 12 or whatever it was, and she immediately told me that I had Alzheimer's disease."

The laughter in the room died as quickly as it had begun.

"'Are you kidding me? I can't draw a clock, and you know I've got Alzheimer's disease? What the hell? That doesn't make sense.' But when somebody tells you you have Alzheimer's disease... you know, that really gets your attention."

Dad continued on with his story, explaining how we sought other medical opinions. "So, I thought I'd go to a real doctor," he said, again lightening the mood by drawing laughter. (Humor had always been a prominent piece of Dad's oratory repertoire—why stop now?) But subsequent diagnoses, including a three-hour-long neuropsychological evaluation, only supported the first. Several weeks later, Dad saw a functional medical doctor who specialized in Alzheimer's. A more complex test administered on a computer left Dad, who never learned to type well and had little experience with a computer (he was an old-school lawyer: papers and dictation), completely flummoxed.

"I go in there and I'm trying to do the test, but I can't type.... I'm in this room for half an hour, and finally the secretary comes in and says, 'Man, are you okay? No one's ever been in here this long.'"

Dad once again has the Rec Center crowd laughing along with his story. His ease with the audience has Mom and me smiling too. He's the same old Dad we've always loved. In flashes, at least.

"She takes me back into the doctor's office," Dad continues, "and he's kind of a smart-ass guy. I sort of liked him."

Nonetheless, the doctor's analysis was clear and concise.

"The first words out of his mouth," Dad told the audience, "were 'You have Alzheimer's disease.' What the hell is with these people? Now I can't work a computer so I have Alzheimer's disease?"

Dad obviously did some time in the denial stage of the grief-and-loss model identified by the work of Swiss-American psychiatrist Elisabeth Kubler-Ross. "I ain't buying it," he told the Rec Center audience. "This can't be me. I'm an athlete. I'm as fit and strong as any 65-year-old person you know." His frustration was palpable, even as he recounted his emotional state of a few weeks earlier. "I could walk right out this door and run 100 miles."

And he could have. No doubt about it. Dad hadn't lost a step on the trail or a pedal stroke on the bike. As in most winters, we had recently traveled together to Leadville, Colorado, to complete 10k snowshoeing races through deep powder at over 10,000 feet in elevation.

But the diagnoses kept stacking up. Anger and frustration followed as Dad tried to process what he was repeatedly hearing—trying to reconcile what he was told he was going to become with what he had always been.

"I thought, I don't deserve this," he told the audience. "Despite the fact that I was a lawyer, I tried to be a good person" (more laughter)... "Tried to take care of my family and my kids... tried to help other people if they needed help. And I thought, This is not fair. But as I kept thinking about it, I thought, Of course it's not fair, but it's not fair to anybody. It's not fair to anyone who has Alzheimer's or cancer or any of that stuff, but I've got to come to grips with it... that it has happened to me. Now I've got to do the best I can."

Dad shared with the crowd the story of how he had waited weeks for an appointment with a neurologist at one of the most prominent hospitals in the state. Even as the reality of Alzheimer's set in, many questions still burned. The functional medicine doctor he'd seen had explained that Alzheimer's has myriad possible causes, among them past head injury, toxic exposure, vascular/heart health, diet, and sleep deprivation. If the causation could be narrowed, maybe we could optimize some kind of treatment regimen. Dad was desperate. We were all desperate. The clock was ticking, and waiting for an appointment was brutal.

I'd heard Dad tell this story plenty of times before, but, no matter, I watched him deliver it to the Rec Center crowd with tears in my eyes.

"I finally get in to see this guy, and after spending ten or fifteen minutes talking to him, he said he wanted me to draw pictures... including a damn clock. And again, I flunked the clock test. In any event, this doctor told me, 'You've got Alzheimer's disease, and you need to get your affairs in order.'"

In front of the room, Dad blinked hard, shook his head once almost imperceptibly, and shifted his weight, his hands in his pockets.

Then something flashed. His expression changed. "This guy looked me right in the eye and said, 'Do as much as you can with the next two or three years.'"

"Well, yeah, bullshit," Dad said, seeming to slip into litigator mode, emphatically poking a finger at an imaginary courtroom adversary. "That guy didn't know me. *Get my affairs in order!* I'm not gettin' my affairs in order! My affairs are now more out of order than they were at the time he told me that, 'cause I ain't doing that."

The audience laughed, but Dad was steely. "I'm not kidding. I swear to God, I'm not doing that. I'm standing there and... my jaw dropped.... I can't even believe that somebody is telling me, in effect, 'You're dying—take a vacation.'"

With his resolve clear and his audience rapt, Dad began his closing argument: his message of hope. He didn't get into the details, but he told the group about our family's recent adoption of the Bredesen Protocol, an individualized treatment regimen for Alzheimer's sufferers created by neurologist Dale Bredesen. The Bredesen Protocol challenged much of the traditional thinking about Alzheimer's, and through customized therapeutic processes (which, in Dad's case included a strict diet and exercise), offered something most rare to Alzheimer's patients—hope of reversal of cognitive decline and possibly even recovery of lost brain function.

"There are some smart people here who are going to explain the Bredesen Protocol to you in more detail," Dad said, referring to Mom and me as the next speakers, "but what I want to tell you before I sit down is that no matter what happens, you've *got* to maintain hope. This protocol may possibly save your life, or my life, or it may stop the advance of this disease. But despite what it may or may not be capable of, you've just got to maintain hope. I'm telling this to you guys because *I* need to maintain hope. I need to make sure that I never give up hope."

Dad looked over at Mom and me frequently during his talk, and even more so now as he wrapped up. Hope is a vague word that has become hackneyed and anemic. It's damnable for what it implies. It's what you have left when your other options have run out. We are active people, at our core, and hope, I think in my lower moments, is a passive word.

But when Dad looked at Mom, he saw real flesh-and-blood evidence of the actual power of hope. He saw the embodiment of hope's triumph over fear, and yes, even over death.

In our family, Dad and I have always been the rivers that run. We are in constant motion. Mom is the rock. Her own health challenges never seemed to diminish her. Not her spirit, anyway. It's hard to summon an unbiased view of your own mother, but Aunt Boo captures Mom's strength and heart when she says: "Pam is the most uplifting and positive person I've ever met. No matter what it is, Pam will find a positive side of it. I've never met anyone like her, someone who's been through what she's been through. [She's] so giving, so loving. There's just unconditional love coming out of her all over the place. And I think that influenced Mark quite a bit—adopting and fostering kids, taking care of them—that brought some hard times, too, but they worked through it together. They never give up on anybody."

Dad told the Rec Center audience the story of Mom's long history of organ failure and transplants (with Mom's help plugging in the key dates), and as he did so, the love and admiration in his eyes as he looked at Mom had the eyes of the audience as wet as my own.

"Pam has been saved *three times* after being told she wouldn't live," Dad said. "'Get your affairs in order,' right? No. She never gave up hope. *We* never gave up hope. That's our family story. I believe in it. And I'm never gonna give up hope. I'm not gonna let this disease get me down. I'm gonna keep doing everything I've always done. I'm not stopping."

Dad's statement felt like the perfect crescendo. But it wasn't just a hollow vow constructed to end the talk on a high note. When Dad said he was going to keep doing everything he'd always done, well, that was saying something. This wasn't like a typical senior citizen saying he or she was going to keep walking the dog every day or keep up with volunteer work at church.

What Dad said next made my eyes widen and my heart rate jump. "The Eco-Challenge adventure race is coming back next year to Fiji," he said. The crowd hung on every word. Many in attendance had watched Dad, Marshall, and their teammates compete internationally in the televised event from 1995 to 2002. "It's an eleven-day race, and I'm going. I don't give a shit. I'm going." The audience broke into spontaneous applause, followed immediately by laughter as he added, "That's if they let us in. You gotta apply for the race... but I'm going and Marshall's going with me."

The lump in my throat almost jumped out. I wanted him to get out there, traveling, racing, being with his tribe. And I wanted to be there as well. But would that even be possible? Was there any chance in the world that ten months from now a sixty-five-year-old with Alzheimer's could be doing an eleven-day, nonstop adventure race in the jungle that included trekking, biking, paddling, navigating, swimming, and canyoneering? I knew Dad had always been a stalwart who put his head down and never looked back, but was competing in one of the hardest races in the world really possible? I mean, hell, even getting to the starting line seemed a bit like magical thinking.

FIVE

I did not treat Pammy very well today. In fact, I treated her horribly and she certainly didn't deserve it…. I still can't get over the fact that I can't drive. I partly blame it on Pammy because she brought it up with the doctor, who recommended I not drive at all. I blame Pammy for taking away my last two miles of independence to drive to the Rec Center and favorite mountain to run. Of course, she's right, but it's not that simple. I've always been independent and taken care of myself, and it appears that at least for the time being, I have to rely upon others and I resent it.

—MACE'S JOURNAL

DAD LOVES HIS FAMILY more than anything, and I knew he truly felt bad about speaking rudely to Mom because she'd brought up driving with the doctor. I also knew they'd get through it because family was always number one for both of them.

In second place, at least for Dad, came his trucks. He really loved the one he was driving at the time of his diagnosis, a 2013 Dodge Ram 1500 with a custom blue-and-tan trim package that he'd spent months picking out. Out here in the West, a man's truck is a tangible symbol of his independence, masculinity, and readiness to get out the door and up a rocky road to do something big.

"That's like shooting me," Dad had told the Rec Center crowd about having his truck keys taken away, as tears again filled his eyes. "It took away my ability to go places on my own."

The first blow had actually come a few months earlier when Dad and Mom had mutually decided to sell the travel trailer they had bought around the time he retired. Like so many retirees, their plan had been to use their well-earned and new-found freedom to explore the country, particularly the West, where there were endless mountain trails to run and adventures to be had. But navigating the twenty-five-foot Cougar travel trailer on winding mountain roads proved too harrowing. Dad's journal entries from around that time make his dejection clear. "I just can't trust myself anymore to pull that trailer," he wrote on October 21, 2018. "I can't even describe how sad I am." Still, he maintained hope. An entry from a few days later reads: "Still thinking about our trailer almost every day.... For me, victory over Alzheimer's disease can be claimed when Pammy and I hit the road in our new trailer."

But if surrendering the trailer brought heartache, giving up the Ram was true heartbreak.

At the time, I was driving a reliable Toyota Tundra that got me and my family all over the Rockies to remote places for racing, camping, skiing, hunting, and fishing, so I wasn't really looking for a different vehicle. But it was clear: Dad was never going to turn *his* truck over to a stranger. We agreed that I'd buy the Ram for whatever amount I got for the Tundra, and soon the deal was done.

Driving home from the DMV with my new truck title on the seat next to me, country music playing as always, I listened closely as Lee Brice's "I Drive Your Truck" came on the radio. It's sung from the perspective of a guy coping with the loss of his brother.

I drive your truck

I roll every window down

And I burn up
Every back road in this town
I find a field, and I tear it up
'Till all the pain's a cloud of dust, yes, sometimes
Brother, sometimes, I drive your truck
I drive your truck
I hope you don't mind,
I hope you don't mind
I drive your truck

I couldn't see through the tears so I pulled off onto a dirt side road, parked the Ram, and cried myself through the end of that song and a few more. As I look at the lyrics now on my computer, it still hits me; tears are on my keyboard.

It took about four months for the Ram to feel like "my" truck. Time passed, my kids and dogs filled the backseat with their stuff, and I put a Northstar truck camper on it so I could camp anytime, anywhere—not only with my wife and kids but also with my dad. I'm just like Dad in many ways, but while he always kept his truck's interior pristine, I think of mine more like a roving locker room, snack shop, kennel, and kidmobile—you get the idea. Most items in the cab don't really have a "place," but there's a special spot reserved under the driver's seat for an old, wrinkled, red stuff sack Dad probably got in the '70s for some winter backpacking trip in Michigan with his college roommate, Ed. That stuff sack has taken its place under each and every one of Dad's truck seats, holding his wallet, pocket knife, and spare Skoal can (Dad finally kicked that old habit about five years ago, and I only dip once a decade or so, just so I can get sick and remember how much I hate it after the quick buzz). I don't know if it was the Alzheimer's or an intentional passing of the torch, but Dad's red stuff sack—the same one I longed for as a kid—came with the Ram. There it stays. Every once in a while, driving down a Colorado highway—say, US 285 where it comes over Kenosha Pass and looks down into South Park onto endless greens, reds, browns, whites, and blues—I reach down and feel that old stuff sack. Sometimes I feel sad, but usually I feel really fucking proud. I drive your truck, Dad. I drive your truck.

The Bredesen Protocol had offered Dad—and all of us—a lifeline. For nearly two months, Dad had adhered to the strict regimen including diet, exercise, and supplements (an amalgam of fifty pills a day) custom-designed for him by the functional medicine doctor and the MD we'd chosen as Dad's primary Alzheimer's caregiver. Dad also endured a near-daily course of photobiomodulation, which uses lower-level laser light and is thought to heal injured or degenerating tissue, including brain tissue. Yes, he would occasionally cheat on the diet—the Thanksgiving and Christmas holidays were particularly hard—but you would be hard-pressed to find a more dedicated adherent to the protocol. We all considered this a life-or-death matter, and we treated it that way.

But the empirical evidence was impossible to ignore. Again, Dad's journal reveals brutal honesty:

> *I am not the same the last couple of weeks.*
> *I'm not laughing or joking like I normally do.*
> *I started the Bredesen Protocol six weeks ago,*
> *and I'm scared because it's not working.*

All of this—the truck, the failing protocol, the uncertainty, the anxiety, the sense of being overwhelmed—left me, as Dr. Seuss said in my favorite book, *Oh, the Places You'll*

Go!, "in a lurch." I'd personally call it a "fucking shitty place," and my search for a way out led me to *Finding Meaning in the Second Half of Life: How to Finally, Really Grow Up*, by Jungian psychoanalyst James Hollis, PhD. The wordy text (some might call it bland, but I love it) engages one (one being me, and hopefully at least a few other persevering readers) for more than eight hours on Audible. I listened to it repeatedly, engaged, inspired, saddened, and enlightened as I drove, skied, ran, and rode.

Hollis called the hole in which I wallowed "the swampland of despair." He didn't really offer a clear way out—I don't know if there ever is one, other than a good run in the woods, which is unfortunately fleeting. But what I really appreciated was the conclusion that undergoing such forced trauma and searching in a dark night of the soul really did serve a purpose. The text showed me that continuing forward, enduring, doing my best (even if that wasn't much at times) could result in one thing alone: growth.

Focusing on growth brought me to Krista Tippett's *On Being* podcast, specifically an episode with guest Pauline Boss about "ambiguous loss." Boss, who wrote *Ambiguous Loss: Learning to Live with Unresolved Grief* and *Loving Someone Who Has Dementia*, identified in her research that ambiguous loss (like that faced by the family of a soldier who is missing in action) is different from loss with closure (like that faced by the family of a soldier who is killed and brought home). Both are terrible, but the grief process is different. With the ambiguous loss—and Boss includes dementia in this category—the stages of grief are more likely to be cyclical and ongoing over time. Did this revelation give me *the answer*? Nope, but it helped me prepare to do my best to hang in there for the long run and to be more accepting of myself when powerful emotions like grief, sadness, and anger came knocking, sometimes unexpectedly. Learning about the ambiguous loss experienced by others helped me realize I wasn't alone. The Macy family was trekking along a tough path, but it was one that had been traveled by people for generations. And, if we looked closely, there were probably others moving along the same challenging route who could become part of our team.

I was going to need all the team I could get because the lows were pretty low. For years I had loved running the picturesque Chimney Gulch Trail, overlooking Denver and Golden to the east and the snow-covered Continental Divide to the west. One morning in March, I dropped the kids at school and drove to the trailhead, seeking the solace I often find in a good, hard session of running, riding, or ski touring. I generally feel especially good on bluebird Colorado days like that one, when the sun shines down on fresh snow on the Ponderosa pines. The Chimney Gulch Trail climbs about 2,000 vertical feet in less than three miles. It's unrelenting, and I like that because it forces me to be present while running, the pain of the ascent temporarily washing away the pain of things that might be bothering me. Turning to run down the trail after summiting, I sought the freedom that often comes with running down a mountain trail, the flow and energy and primal wildness of running through the woods on strong legs over rocky terrain. I think it's a feeling humans were made to experience, and I wish more of them could or would.

A few minutes later, though, I found myself literally struggling to breathe. Worries about Alzheimer's had come crashing back into my awareness like the avalanches that had ripped through the Colorado high country that week: a thump, a crack, a rumble, a roar. Tumbling in a suffocating cascade of emotions, my thoughts raced: where we were with the disease at the moment, future hypotheticals that might come, complete dismay about who I could turn to when the one person I always turned to might slowly slip away. As I sobbed in a panic, literally gasping for air as I staggered down the trail, I racked my brain for some way to escape.

No escape appeared, so I just kept running.

Running has always been an escape for me. Running, trekking, pedaling, paddling— pushing my body has always been balm to my soul. Dad and I are not all that different from anyone else physiologically: we've got the same body parts and functionality, even if ours and those of other endurance athletes are optimized to our athletic pursuits. The difference, I believe, ultimately comes down to will—the will to overcome the odds, the suffering, doubt, fear... the sheer will to not accept an alternative outcome.

But this was different. The Bredesen Protocol wasn't working. The endless hours spent online searching for alternative approaches—searching for a lifeline—were not working. I am exhausted. Exhausted from running after glimmers of hope, researching clinical trials, chasing dead ends. Momentary hope followed by frustration and despair.

Will isn't enough. Faith seems foolish. This disease is immutable. It doesn't care. It doesn't care if you are a good person who has helped others your entire life. A person who adopted and fostered children in an effort to give them a shot at a life with better prospects. The kind of person who would donate an organ to save the life of a stranger. Alzheimer's doesn't give a shit.

This is powerlessness, by definition. Fate is locked in. Will is meaningless. Which leaves, what? Despair, self-pity, preemptive grief? Is there really nothing more than the long, slow good-bye?

I often found myself walking the dogs for hours in the cold and wintry night, sometimes calmed by the frigid air on my face and other times with my eyes on fire from wiping tears. Amy and I have, thankfully, not lost any of our parents, and this new experience with mortality—my dad's, which made me think about my own—strained our relationship. People who've gone around the block in challenging sports like adventure racing and ultrarunning can't help but learn that often the most important things in life are also the hardest. I don't know about you, but Amy and I find that to be true about marriage and parenting. No relationship is perfect, and even the great ones bring unresolvable challenges. In many contemporary families with young children, including ours, both parents work. Strains on time and energy are almost constant, and it's tough for spouses to find time to connect with each other. To this backdrop was now added the new stress of Alzheimer's, including my own neediness for connection (ideally through what some might call "conjugal intimacy") on the one hand and lots of time away on the other—time to be with Dad *and* time to release and escape through training, hunting, and hanging with the guys.

So how do you make it to the end of a dark tunnel that doesn't end? It's a great question, and my best answer is probably, "Just keep going." Jung said, "The greatest and most important problems of life are all fundamentally insoluble. They can never be solved but only outgrown." I realized I had no choice but to hang in there, one day, one minute, one mile at a time. For me, and for Dad, to "keep going" means to lace up your damn shoes and do what you do. That means we run. We ride. We climb. We trek. We swim. We fight. We don't hold on and wait for a miracle. We work. We *move*.

No doubt about it, that first winter after the diagnosis was brutal, but we were adapting to the new reality—all of us were. It was during these daylight-deprived winter days that I learned my first Alzheimer's lessons: Life is actually a lot less under your control than you imagined or wanted it to be. Instead of absolutes there are lots of in-betweens, gray areas, times to push and times to ease up. Times to be determined and times to change your mind. I've got to become more comfortable with long-term uncertainty. Interestingly, these lessons go hand in hand with ultraendurance racing, which by necessity involves many variables we can't control.

At higher moments, I found inspiration in Hollis's writing about Jung's "second half of life," which might be reached through struggle and despair, and might (I hoped) result in a deeper peace and individuation and sincere focus on generating positive impact. So, here I am, writing this book. The Macy family has found some peace and acceptance with this Alzheimer's thing, but let me be clear: it's still really hard. My current silver lining as I explore my own second half of life is this: I hope this book helps you.

And one more takeaway: If the overriding message of my previous book, *The Ultra Mindset,* says, "Just keep hammering and things will be okay," this book says, "Keep hammering but also pump the brakes and get creative and ask for help. Maybe even call the tow truck at times."

I used to be able to take care of myself. I used to go to Alaska to race a hundred miles on snowshoes on the Iditarod trail. I enjoyed the solitude of being out there alone, in the dark, with the Northern Lights and the wolves. Sure, I got lost sometimes; good and lost. But then in the good old days I knew I could find my way

*out. Now I'm awake for hours the night before a
ten-mile race because I'm afraid I'll get lost.*

—MACE'S JOURNAL

One of my favorite things about adventure racing is
that it's a team sport—and that it can teach you about life
because life is also a team sport. It became clear early in
our Alzheimer's journey that a team-oriented approach was
the only option for us. Each of us would need to look for
opportunities to give help and to ask for help. We'd need to
become comfortable in these roles. It might not be easy for
Dad to accept that he needed help with driving, finances,
technology, and planning. It might not be easy for me to
accept that overwhelming anxiety and depression necessi-
tated medication and therapy. Anxiety and depression had
been on my radar for awhile, especially since a concussion
sustained while body surfing a few years earlier. Our family
history includes significant alcoholism, and when I noticed
an uncomfortable increase in my own reliance on the bottle,
I decided ongoing therapy and medication were a better alternative. I don't like to talk too much about which medications
have helped me because I know different options work for
different people (and I'm not a doctor), but I can say this: If
you think you might benefit from help, please get it. Mental
health is a priority that, for me, necessitates an all-hands-on-
deck approach. End the stigma and talk about mental health.
Take active steps so you can be happy and be your best for
yourself and your community.

Nope, not easy for Dad or me to ask for and accept help,
but we had to put our egos aside and "take one for the team,"
as it were. Comfort with vulnerability is essential in so many
areas of life. Here, it really helped us shift the stories we

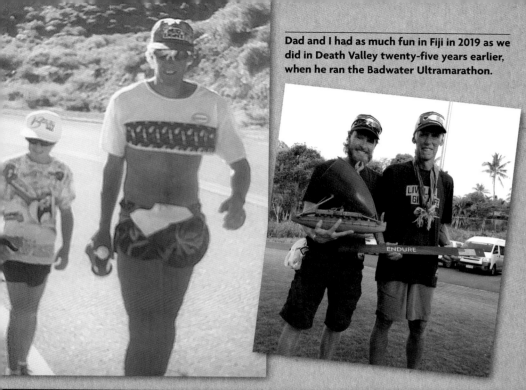

Dad and I had as much fun in Fiji in 2019 as we did in Death Valley twenty-five years earlier, when he ran the Badwater Ultramarathon.

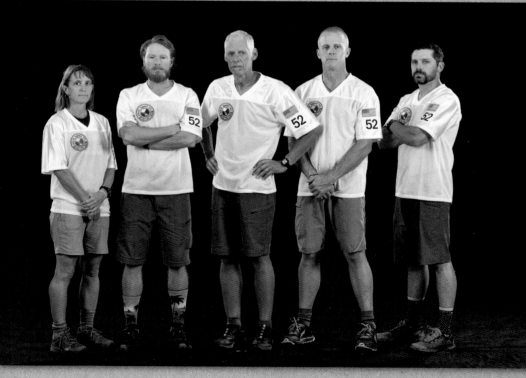

Left to right: Danelle Ballengee, me, Dad, Shane Sigle, and Andrew Speers at the World's Toughest Race. They told us to "look tough."

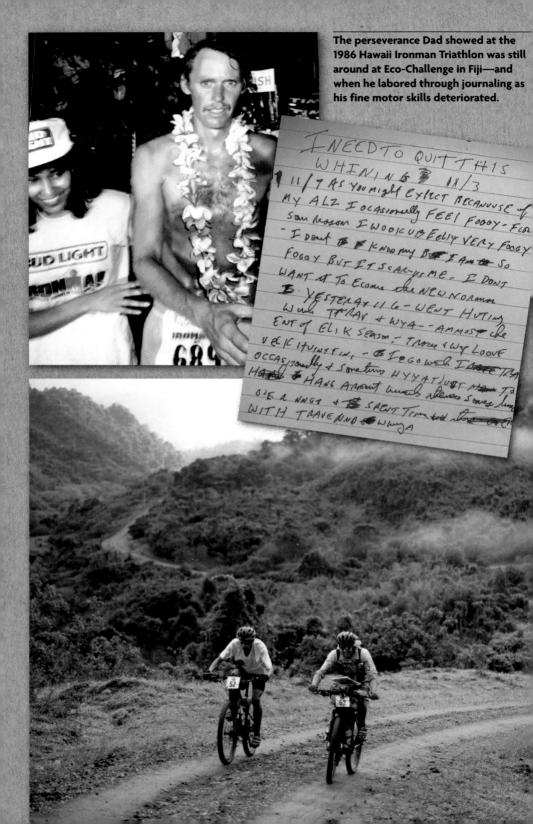

The perseverance Dad showed at the 1986 Hawaii Ironman Triathlon was still around at Eco-Challenge in Fiji—and when he labored through journaling as his fine motor skills deteriorated.

The Eco-Challenge started with a long journey in traditional Fijian *camakau* outrigger canoes.

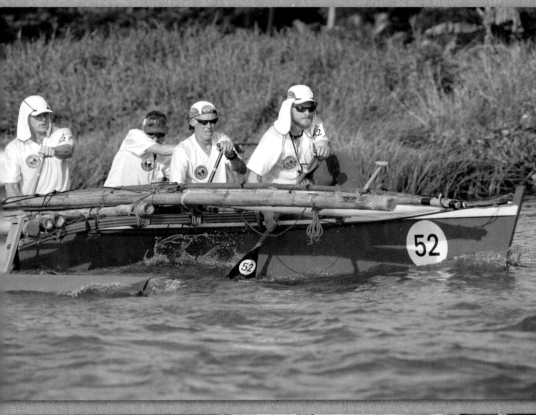

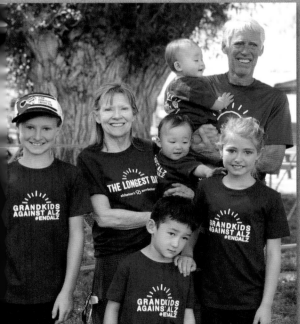

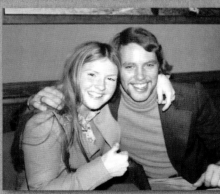

Mom and Dad have always been a team—from high school to now, when they're incredible grandparents.

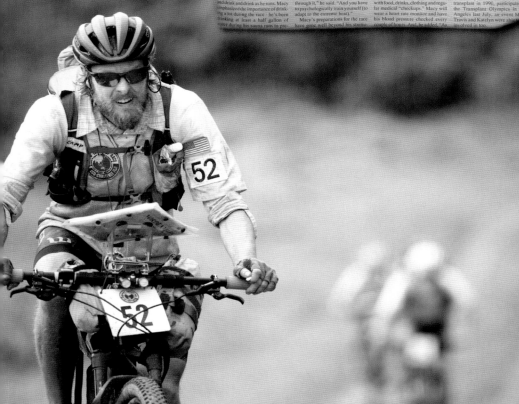

Adventure racing is hard, but like Dad, I've always loved being out there.

People

by Ann Morris
Associate Editor

Anyone who's been hanging out in the Evergreen Fitness and Racquet Club's sauna lately may have noticed a peculiar scene - a guy running in place, sweating his heart out and drinking about as much water as his body could handle. No, he's not doing it just for kicks. He's actually been preparing for a race, a race where he'll be in much tougher conditions than the sweltering 180-degree heat of the club's sauna.

Evergreen resident Mark Macy is one of about 20 runners from around the country invited to participate in the upcoming Badwater 146, a grueling 146-mile race in Death Valley, Calif. The runners will not only be facing 120-degree temperatures (90- to 100-degree temps at night) but they'll also be running from the lowest point in the lower United States (282 feet below sea level) to the summit of Mount Whitney, which, at 14,494 feet above sea level, is the highest point in the lower United States.

Macy, a Denver attorney, has been running since 1984 and has participated in his share of races, but he's never been in a race equal to the Badwater 146. To prepare for it, he's been running 10 to 15 miles a day during the week and 20 to 50 miles a day on weekends. This on top of his 45-minute runs in the Evergreen Fitness and Racquet Club's sauna.

Macy said he hopes to complete the Badwater 146 in 48 hours, stopping for only an hour or two after the first 130 miles. He'll eat and drink and drink and drink as he runs. Macy emphasized the importance of drinking a lot during the race - he's been drinking at least a half gallon of water during his sauna runs to prepare his body to accept the enormous amount of fluids he'll drink during the race.

"What you've got to do is you've got to train your body to be able to handle that much water running through it," he said. "And you have to psychologically train yourself (to adapt to the extreme heat)."

Macy's preparations for the race have gone well beyond his strenuous workouts. He's arranged for a crew to accompany him along every mile of the race. His crew, which will consist of his wife Pam and friends Don Gautier, Tim Graim and Dale Peterson, will provide him with food, drinks, clothing and regular medical "checkups." Macy will wear a heart rate monitor and have his blood pressure checked every couple of hours. And, he added, "As

silly as it sounds, they'll have to keep track of how often I'm urinating to make sure my system's still working."

Macy's crew will also carry five to six extra pairs of running shoes. With road temperatures in the 180- to 200-degree level, his shoes will melt and need to be replaced periodically.

Aside from his crew, Macy has a number of sponsors supporting him for the race, including Runner's Roost in Denver, Nike, Exceed, which provides nutritional food and drink, and the Evergreen Fitness and Racquet Club.

Though the Badwater 146 will be a major race for Macy, it's still just one of many he'll do throughout the year. "I do several triathlons a year and I'll do several this year," he said. "I probably do two or three other ultra-marathons a year and that's anything over 26 miles. And I do some winter triathlon-type races.

Of the three events in a triathlon - running, biking and swimming - Macy said he thinks running is the most challenging "because it's always last so you're always tired."

Macy and his wife Pam are going to make the Badwater 146 a family affair, bringing along their two children, Travis, 10 and Katelyn, 8. The race will no doubt be reminiscent of another athletic event the whole family participated in only a year ago. Pam Macy, who underwent a liver transplant in 1996, participated in the Transplant Olympics in Los Angeles last July, an event Mark, Travis and Katelyn were able to be involved in too.

Mark Macy   Photo provided courtesy Mark Macy

Running to extremes

Evergreen resident Mark Macy is preparing for the Badwater 146, a race that will take him from the lowest point in the U.S. to the highest.

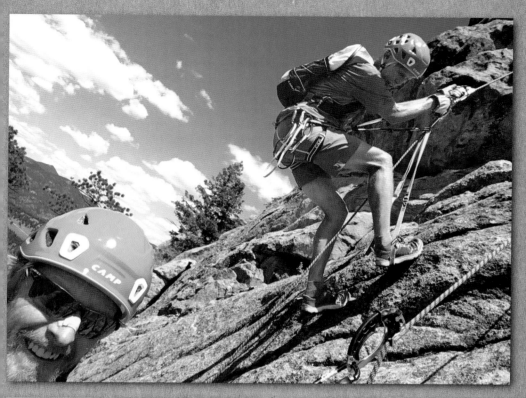

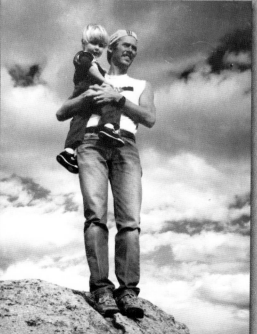

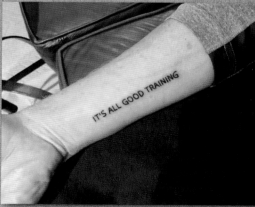

Dad's first tattoo, which he got at age sixty-eight, sums up a life of dedication.

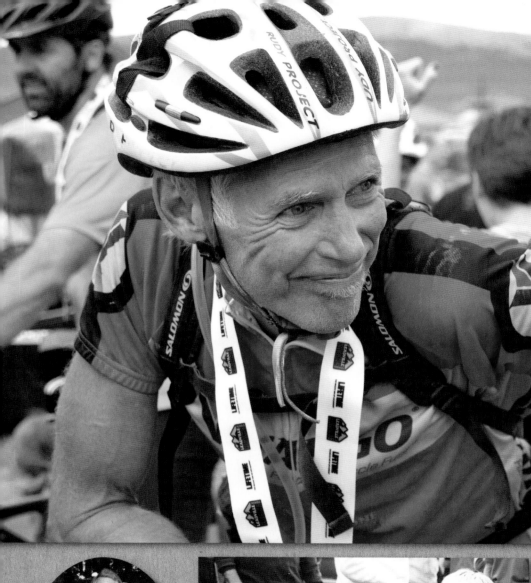

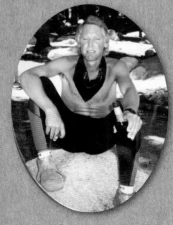

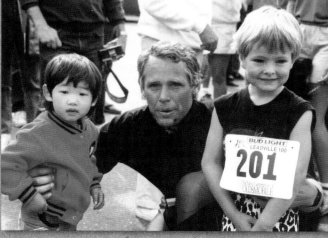

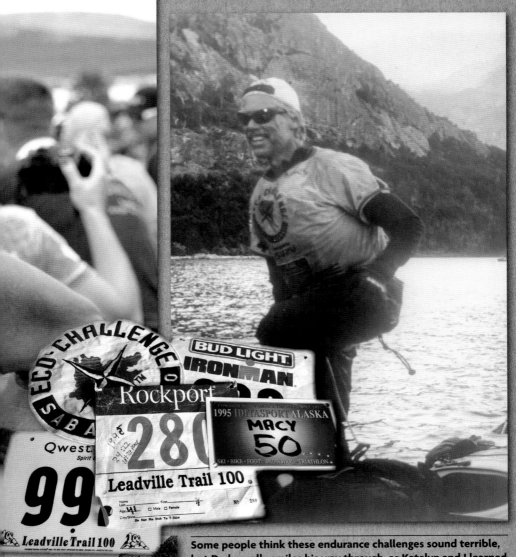

Some people think these endurance challenges sound terrible, but Dad usually smiles his way through, as Katelyn and I learned from an early age.

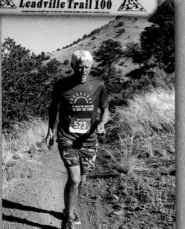

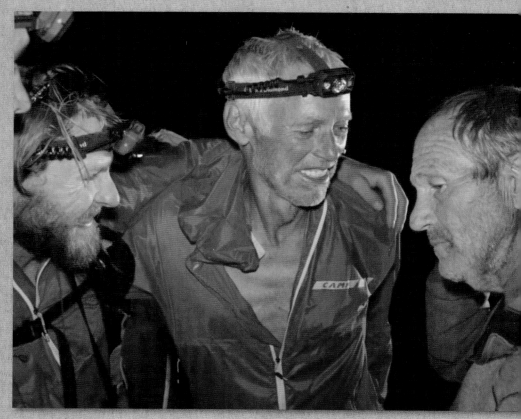

Endurance racing generates powerful relationships, like ours with Marshall Ulrich (above, with Dad and me after the Fiji race), and with our late friend, the great Emma Roca, seen here shaking hands with the host of the race, Bear Grylls.

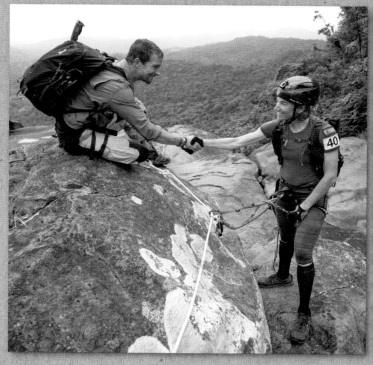

It's a family affair: Dad with Mom's brothers, Eric and Brian Pence, both ultrarunners.

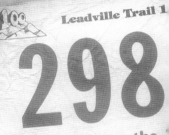

Certificate of Achievement

This Certifies That

Mark Macy

Has completed the
Leadville Trail 100

Place Overall   253
Age Group   61 M4
Time   10.30.06

Race Director
Date   August 14, 1999

Leadville Trail 1

298

The Race Across the

Dad's thirst for adventure took him to the Mountain Man Winter Triathlon (ski, snowshoe, speed skate) many times in the 1980s.

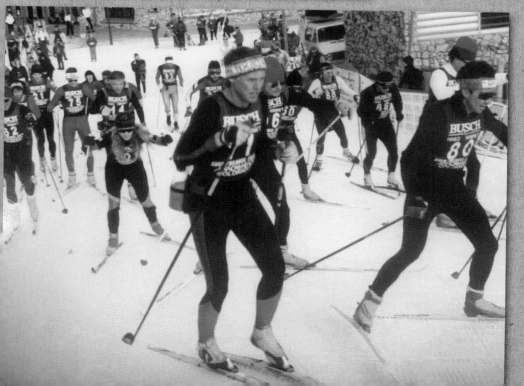

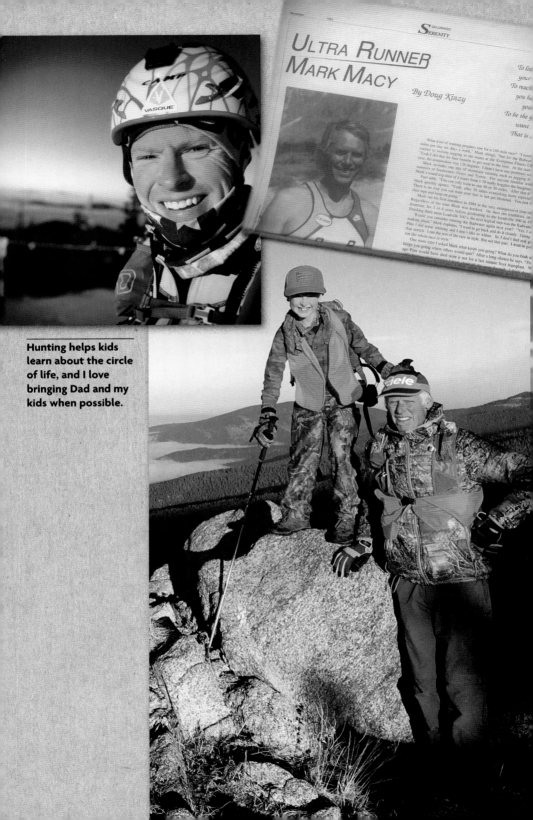

COLORADO
SERENITY

ULTRA RUNNER
MARK MACY

By Doug Kinzy

Hunting helps kids learn about the circle of life, and I love bringing Dad and my kids when possible.

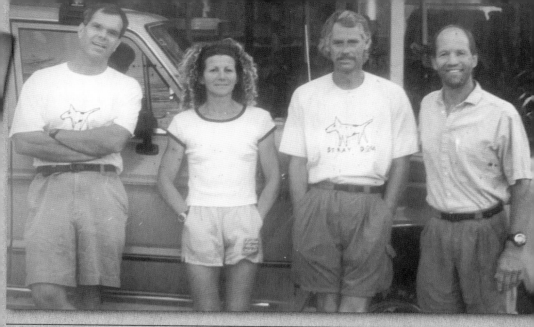

Team Stray Dogs at Eco-Challenge Australia in 1997. Left to right: Dr. Bob Haugh, Sharon "Shaz" Davis, Dad, and Marshall Ulrich.

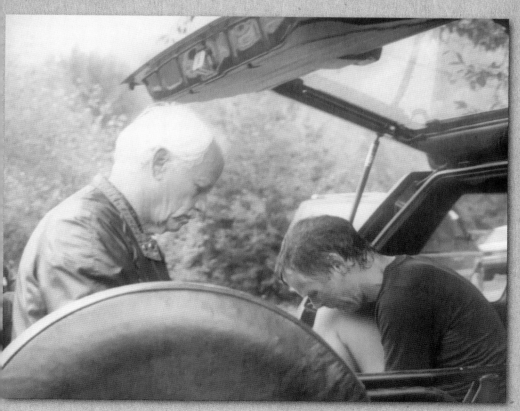

Dad's father, Jack Macy, was one hell of a guy. Compared to the hardship of the front lines in World War II, crewing for Dad all night at ultraruns was probably a piece of cake.

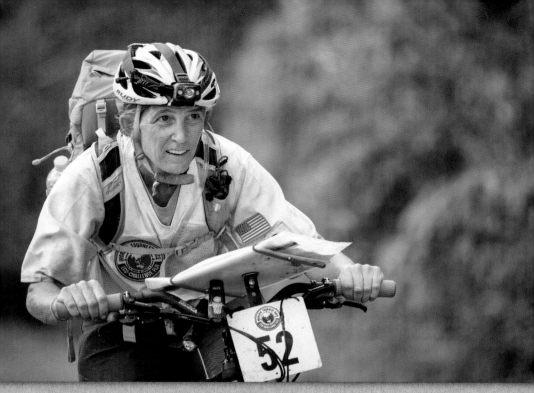

Danelle Ballengee is a loyal friend, committed teammate, and probably the most accomplished athlete you've never heard of.

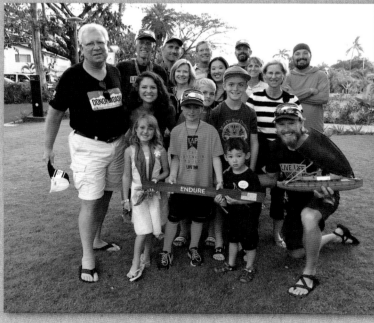

Sharing the postrace festivities in Fiji with our families was special.

The kids of the Macy household in 1995: Keegan, Katelyn, Dona, Haven, and me.

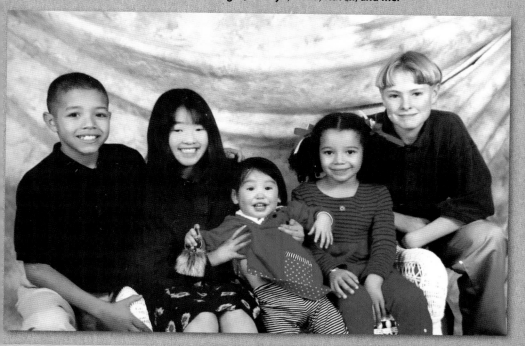

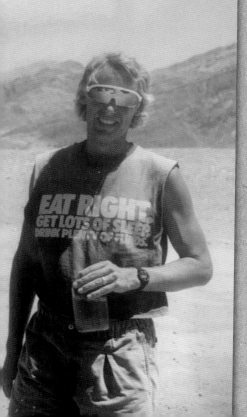

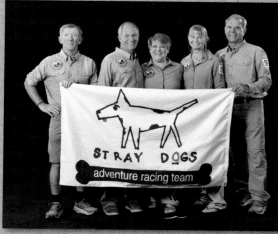

The Stray Dogs in 2019—Dr. Bob and Marshall along with Adrian Crane (left), Heather Ulrich (middle), and Nancy Bristow (second from right)

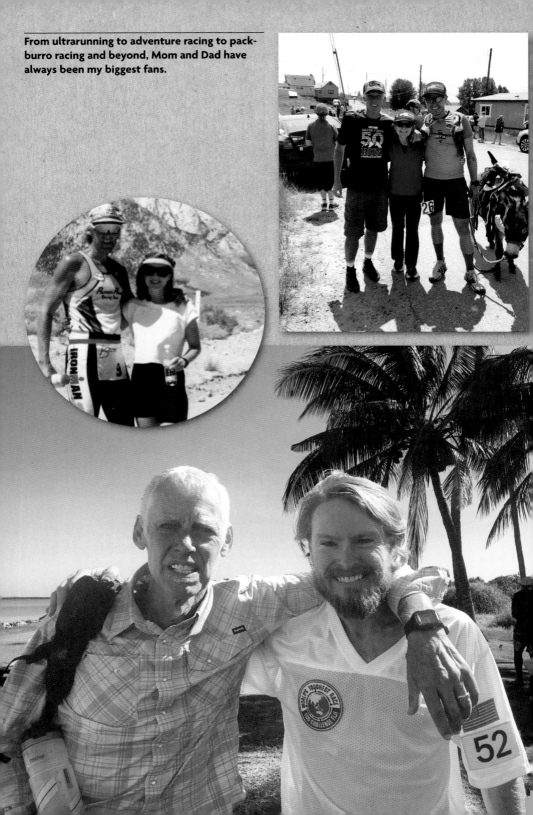

From ultrarunning to adventure racing to pack-burro racing and beyond, Mom and Dad have always been my biggest fans.

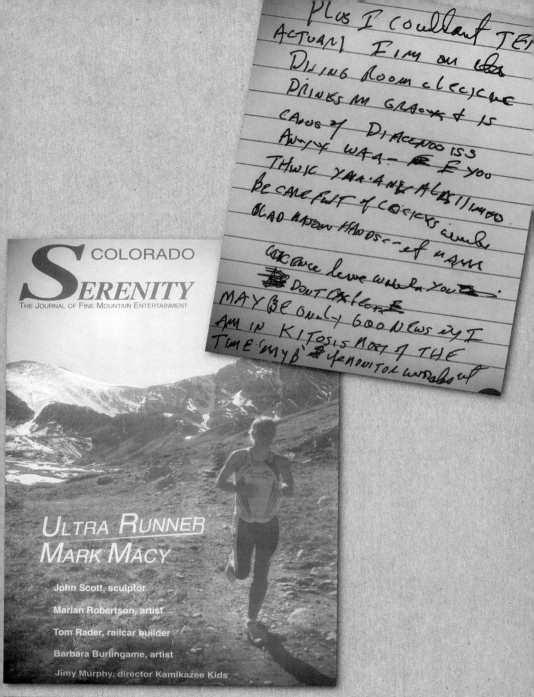

Dad continues to seek serenity by taking on huge challenges.

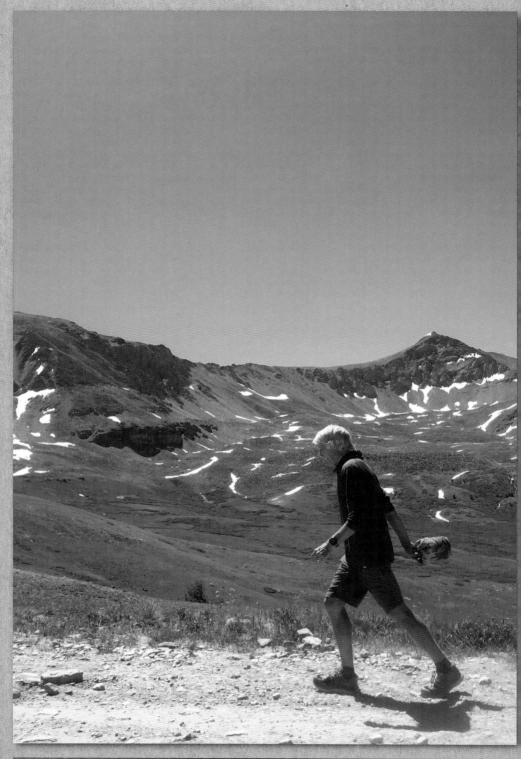

We don't know what's ahead, but we'll keep trekking with Dad...a mile at a time.

told ourselves. Dad went from something like "I can't even drive anymore" (deficit-focused) to "I might as well accept a ride to the Rec Center so I can stay strong and energetic for my grandkids" (strengths-focused and team-oriented). I went from something like "I need mental health medication because I am broken" (all-or-nothing, lacking wisdom) to "If setting my ego aside to take a pill makes me a better person for my family and allows me to get through something hard and inherently out of my control, then let's give it a shot" (nuanced, curious, generous).

As the Rocky Mountain winter melted into spring, our team-based approach held strong. Even as I looked to books, lectures, and wise friends for reassurance, the greatest inspiration in keeping it together was Mom. As I said, she is the rock in our family. For months, Mom and I had been attending a support group for Alzheimer's caregivers, but as the weeks passed, an unspoken dissatisfaction had crept in. One night in March, Mom called and said she was finished with the group. It was overly focused on deficits, losses, and problems and not enough on the remaining strengths that could empower Alzheimer's sufferers and their loved ones. I agreed completely. I had learned this lesson time and again in team sports including adventure racing: energy, be it positive or negative, is contagious. Despite the support group's admirable intentions, Mom and I weren't getting the right kind of energy from being a part of it. We decided to double down on our own group instead.

In addition to therapists and family members, I sought support from a wide range of friends. Mark Livingston and I became friends when I coached him through the Leadman series a few years earlier. His mother has Alzheimer's, and conversations with Mark about logistics and planning proved very helpful for me. Similarly, Mom and I made a serendipitous connection through an Alzheimer's Association meet-up in our small town. We noticed in that roundtable conversation an older woman with energy and spark who, while acknowledging the hardship of the disease, seemed to focus on the positives: what folks still *could* do; how their caregivers might continue leading their own lives; support systems and teams that should be employed to give spouses a break. Her contagious enthusiasm was immediately familiar, and I soon realized why. Sue Pyle, it turns out, was the same Mrs. Pyle who had taught first grade at Wilmot Elementary in the '80s when my sister Katelyn and I were there! Long since retired from classroom teaching, Sue was still fully engaged in making the world a better place, now by teaching families impacted by dementia to navigate the journey with a sense of optimism. Sue's street cred came from caring for her own father through Alzheimer's and then her husband through vascular dementia; she wasn't sugarcoating the challenges. Yet there was a spark, a sense that things really could be okay if a family hung in there together. In *The Ultra Mindset*, I wrote about a concept called "Be a Wannabe." The idea is that we should identify people we'd like to emulate in one way or another and try to learn from them. Well, I'm not ashamed to say that I want to be like Mrs. Pyle.

My anxiety about World's Toughest Race remained high as spring became summer and the September race grew near. Yes, I was excited, but also uncertain about the wisdom of combining Alzheimer's with one of the toughest races in the world—especially since Dad's prospective teammates were all in their sixties as well.

Team Stray Dogs developed a legendary status in adventure

racing in the 1990s. They didn't do it by winning but simply by showing up. And then showing up again and again. I think there's something to be said for Woody Allen's idea that 80 percent of success is just showing up; Dad and his teammates set the example here. As *Mark Burnett's Eco-Challenge,* one of the original reality TV shows and a cult hit of the era, moved from Utah to British Columbia, Argentina, Morocco, Australia, New Zealand, Borneo, and Fiji, these guys kept showing up, finishing the races, smiling as they toughed it out, and helping other teams do the same.

Dad met Marshall Ulrich through ultrarunning in the early 1990s. Marsh was, at the time, one of the best ultra-runners in the world, having won the Badwater Ultramarathon (135 miles across Death Valley to the summit of Mt. Whitney) numerous times. Dad and I followed closely as Marsh, who lived nearby in Colorado, went on to climb the Seven Summits, run across America, and complete many other incredible races and journeys. When Dad and Marsh took me on a run up Grays Peak, a local 14,000-ft. peak, during my freshman year of high school, I remember thinking at the summit, Damn, I just ran up a mountain with Marshall Ulrich! I can do anything now! In 2019, as World's Toughest Race approached, Marsh and his wonderful wife, Heather, lived in Evergreen. They had become a key piece of our Alzheimer's support team and brought incredible energy to the process of preparing for Fiji, Heather often leading the way with the endless research and organization of gear, certifications, and other necessary details.

Dad's other prospective teammates on Stray Dogs are also highly experienced athletes. Adrian Crane is a master navigator with map and compass whose resume includes numerous adventure racing and mountaineering feats, including the *Guinness Book of World Records* high-altitude bicycling record (20,300 feet) on Mt. Chimborazo in Ecuador. Nancy Bristow has completed over a hundred triathlons in addition to many adventure races and international mountaineering expeditions. Dr. Bob Haugh, one of the most personable folks I've known, is a retired pathologist who consistently finishes adventure races and ultraruns. Dr. Bob may not have a whole lot of talent or the skinny body of the typical endurance athlete (he was a linebacker in college at the University of Kentucky), but when it comes to grit, determination, perspective, and humor, he's second to none.

Team Stray Dogs' plan was for Dad to race with Marsh, Adrian, and Nancy while Dr. Bob acted as Team Assistance Crew (TAC; driving from camp to camp in the race and supporting the team with gear, food, first aid, and encouragement). This was truly one of the most experienced teams in the world. That said, they were all born in the 1950s, which didn't sound that long ago to them but did to me. We knew Eco would push any athlete to his or her limit; it would be especially hard for folks over sixty. Even if they were some of the most experienced athletes around, would the Stray Dogs be able to persevere through the course while navigating the additional unknown challenges presented by Alzheimer's?

I had simultaneously gathered my own team for the event, and we were thinking about making a bid for the podium. We had applied as Team Colorado by submitting a written application and team video. Eco-Challenge is a real race, but it was also being produced for a ten-episode series on Amazon Prime, so charisma on camera was probably one of the selection criteria. I had teamed with Erik Sanders and Jari Hiatt, both former teammates who are fit, fast, and fun. Erik and I had enjoyed teaming up in the Elk Mountains Grand Traverse, a forty-mile, overnight backcountry ski race in Colorado. Jari had led our adventure racing team in years past through big races in Scotland, South Dakota, and Montana. Now a new mom, Jari was excited to get back to elite racing. I was pumped to race with both of them!

In a video call interview for the application process, the screener asked us, "So, what makes your team different?" We hesitated and looked at each other in the corners of our laptops. "Well," chimed in our fourth teammate, Dave Mackey, "we have a guy with one leg."

Dave and I began adventure racing together as I completed college at CU-Boulder in the early 2000s. We became close friends while racing internationally with a team sponsored by Spyder, and I deeply appreciated Dave's quiet hard work and tenacity on the course. In 2015, a fall while mountain running near Boulder left Dave's lower leg injured badly; after many surgeries he elected for a below-the-knee amputation in 2016. Dave had since run a hundred miles in less than twenty-five hours (a very solid time for anyone!) and was ready to race on a prosthetic in Fiji.

Ready, that is, until real life called. Like most elite endurance athletes, Dave balances training and racing with work and family. The coming fall would mean school for Dave's wife (a teacher) and kids, soccer coaching for Dave, and his own demanding job as a physician assistant. Obligation trumped fun, and Dave was out for this edition of Eco-Challenge.

With Team Colorado down to three, Jari, Erik, and I had some thinking to do. Looking within, I discovered my greatest motivation for racing in Fiji: Dad. Of all the races Dad had done when I was a kid, Eco-Challenge left the deepest mark on me; *this* was the race I wanted to do *alongside* my dad. I knew that meant setting competitive goals aside, which was fine with me; sometimes you really do have just one shot to give something a go in a certain way, and I recognized the urgency. So did Erik and Jari. Even though they wanted to compete for the podium and couldn't leave home for three weeks (Erik from his new job and Jari from her new baby) if they didn't have a shot at prize money, they both supported my desire to honor family and experience over competition. And in case it's not clear, I am forever grateful, Jari and Erik.

Racing with Dad was an exhilarating notion, but the voice in my head at 3:00 a.m. had its own ideas: Are you *insane*? Isn't this irresponsible? What are you proving? Who is this serving? Is this ego-driven? Is this the best thing for Dad? For our family?

As I struggled with the decision, I sought advice from some trusted friends.

Tim Weber is an orthopedic surgeon in Indianapolis and a former ultrarunning coaching client. When I shared my quandary with Tim, his reply was compelling: "I work with a lot of older folks, Travis, and the ones who receive an injury or diagnosis and say 'I'm done' usually don't live much longer. But the ones who stay engaged with what they love to do often live a long time and remain happy." Hearing that from a doctor helped me believe that going to the race was actually a responsible thing to do.

Jim Harshaw is a former elite wrestler and executive life coach. When I told him about being accepted for Eco and explained the decision I faced about Dad, he responded with his typical high energy. "Man, congrats on getting in! You've got to be pumped! Your dad's grandkids are going to love watching this on TV!" Jim's outright enthusiasm and cut-to-the-chase approach in pointing out the value of a TV production that could become part of the "family photo album" (especially for the younger grandkids who might not remember Grandpa in his prime) was pretty hard to argue with.

Another friend, Jesse Mattner, the owner of CAMP-USA and a highly experienced mountaineer, adventure racer, and outdoorsman, made it a trifecta. When I told him we got into the race, he seemed to know intuitively this was a once-in-a-lifetime opportunity that should not be missed. He didn't say he was jealous, but I sensed a longing for such adventure, the kind that makes guys who are wired like me and Jesse and Dad tick at a primal level. Dad was already fighting for his life. But what's the point of life if you cease to live it on your terms?

I'd thought about it enough. In May 2019 I called Dad from a family road trip, pausing between casts as I fly-fished the Arkansas River with my eight-year-old son, Wyatt, and six-year-old daughter, Lila. "Hey, Dad, want to do Eco-Challenge with my team?"

"Hell, yeah, I do, Bud! But... what about Stray Dogs? I think they're counting on me, and I can't let them down."

"I think we can figure that out, Dad, and I bet you might even help out an old friend."

In truth, I had already talked with Marsh and Heather. The plan was this: Dad would join me under a new team name, Team Endure, while Dr. Bob competed with Stray Dogs and Marsh's wife, Heather, took on the TAC role for the team. Smart and capable, Heather is detail-oriented and persevering, so she'd be a real asset.

With Erik and Jari stepping back to support the revised team mission, Dad and I needed a couple of teammates. And we knew just who to call.

"Hey, Nellie, how are you?" I was calling from beside the evening campfire on the same family trip. She was doing well in Moab, Utah: raising the kids; training here and there; running her businesses; coaching soccer and basketball; and checking in on her elderly neighbor, who also happened to have Alzheimer's.

"So, do you want to do Eco-Challenge with Dad and me?"

"Well, it has been a while since I did a big adventure race..."

And indeed it had. Danelle "Nellie" Ballengee grew up in my hometown of Evergreen, Colorado, where she excelled as an athlete before becoming (as I did a decade later) a varsity collegiate distance runner and triathlete at CU-Boulder. As a professional endurance athlete over the next decade and a half, Nellie won dozens and dozens of local, domestic, and international races in running, duathlon, triathlon, quadrathlon, snowshoeing, and adventure racing (just to name a few). Many times a national and world champion, Nellie was racing professionally with Dave Mackey and me on Team Spyder when she nearly died in a 2006 training accident that left her pelvis shattered and internal organs damaged. After spending months in a wheelchair and rehab, Nellie had focused on family and business since then, directing her own races and training/competing for the joy of the experience. A true and caring friend who's also tough as nails, Nellie could be a huge asset to Team Endure. I also liked that going to Fiji would give her a chance to fully rebound from a devastating accident and toe the line in the same event in which her team finished second in 2002. Nellie was interested and said she'd get back to me after looking at the work calendar and making sure her kids and their father, B. C. Laprade, could potentially join in Fiji (which was great because Dad and I also wanted our family to make the trip).

In the meantime, I rang another prospective teammate.

"Trav! How ya been!" Shane Sigle and I had immediately developed a close friendship when we met at a race in Brazil in 2005 because we're both stoked by enthusiasm and optimism. Two years later, Amy and I slept on Shane's couch on and off for months as we bummed around

New Zealand, where he lived at the time. And in 2013 he jammed those Cheetos down my throat in Leadville. Now a Durango, Colorado, whitewater engineer (the guy designs kayak parks for a living!) who also grew up in—you guessed it—Evergreen, Shane is a super-experienced elite adventure racer and whitewater paddler. His team led the race for most of Eco-Challenge Fiji 2002 before succumbing, like many teams, to severe foot infection. Shane knew how tough Fiji was—and he knew he was one of a small number of physically and personally suitable people who could contribute to our unique team in just the right ways. Shane was highly interested but also needed a few days to make sure it would work with family and business.

We didn't have to wait long.

"Dad," this time I was back in Evergreen and we were trekking up a mountain trail to prepare for Fiji, "Shane and Nellie are in! And my friend Andrew Speers—you remember, I taught with him at Evergreen High School and he's a really good bike mechanic—is in for support crew."

"All right, Bud! They're all great people. Let's do this."

Team Endure was ready to roll. We knew the challenge was epic. Even more, we believed in ourselves and believed in each other. But before kicking training into high gear, we had one not-insignificant hurdle to clear.

Both Dad's team, the Stray Dogs, and my own Team Colorado had been accepted to participate in Eco-Challenge Fiji. The newly formed Team Endure had not. Race organizers had strict prohibitions against changing the makeup of a team after the field was set. We would need to make an appeal to swap out a member of Stray Dogs *and* replace Team Colorado with a new team made up of 75 percent new members. What's more, one of those members had early-onset Alzheimer's. This would need to be done delicately.

Race organizers were extremely supportive from the start. I wrote to Lisa Hennessy, an executive producer who knew Dad well because she'd worked with Burnett on the early Eco-Challenges. Lisa was in favor of us getting to the race; moreover, she was helpful as a caring and empathetic friend. I think Lisa knew how important getting to Fiji was for our family—regardless of whether or not it would turn out to be a good story on TV. Race director Kevin Hodder was also very receptive, taking the time to talk through various hypotheticals with me to make sure we were on the same page regarding safety.

The barrier, somewhat ironically, would be the lawyers. As a retired attorney, Dad knew well the challenges in navigating potential liability issues. And because the race was backed by Amazon for production as a ten-episode Amazon Prime series, the producers had to pass the buck to a corporate legal team. This made sense and we knew consideration was appropriate. Nonetheless, as the waiting went on and on and on, Dad became impatient: "What the hell are these damn lawyers doing! Why are they taking so long to make a simple decision? I bet they're out having lunch at some fancy restaurant right now!" Some of this was hyperbole and humor, but Dad wasn't exactly a fan of everyone in his previous profession, and we were all ready to get on with official planning for the race, including details like purchasing plane tickets (which were continually going up in price).

In the meantime, our Alzheimer's journey got a nice boost at America's highest road-running race. The Mount Evans Ascent road-running race starts at 10,600 feet near Echo Lake, Colorado, and goes 14.5 miles along the country's highest paved auto road to the summit at 14,264 feet. It's pretty epic running past the mountain goats that often hang out near the road up high, and my best time was just over two hours when I was in college. It had snowed that year, as usual, and Nellie had been the race director. In 2019 we weren't going for records, which was good because the course had to be altered at the last minute when a truck carrying race items slid into the ditch while navigating ice on the road (in June!). Nope, instead of racing all out, a large group of friends gathered to celebrate "Team Mace."

Marsh drove up from his house and Dr. Bob flew in from Kentucky—nothing like going from sea level to above tree line overnight! My high school cross-country coach, Rob Wright, was there, stoked as always to pump up the team with his whoopin' and hollerin'. Longtime friend James Kovacs, PhD, an accomplished science professor and endurance athlete who often provided cutting-edge advice on medical issues came along; if we had any questions, James surely had the answers. Dave Mackey, who braved the black ice with his prosthetic, joined Denver orthopedic surgeon Mike Hewitt to complete the course twice that day for a nice, long "training run." It was a year before COVID (talk about another uncertainty-laden challenge that took us all by surprise!), but Dave and Mike looked like bank robbers with neck scarves up to their eyes in an effort to stave off the biting mountain wind. From start to finish, the whole day was a blast: dark, cold beginning; epic suffering plus constant joking; everyone contributing and traveling as a team; BBQ sandwiches in the sun at the finish. We had a blast, and getting out there for a challenge was a good reminder of how much we wanted to experience an even bigger challenge in Fiji.

By the end of June, we still hadn't heard back from Amazon Legal. Earlier in the spring, I had asked Dad, "If you could go anywhere, where would you go?" He hadn't hesitated: "Alaska, Bud. With you and Wyatt." I didn't hesitate either; flights, rental camper, and fishing guides were soon booked. Dad had been there plenty of times before to compete in snowshoe races and other endurance events. And Alaska held cherished memories for me as well—both from the summer-long childhood Airstream adventure in 1994 and the rite-of-passage post–high school graduation trip with Dad seven years later. Alaska was special, and this trip would be even more so as we'd be taking along my own eight-year-old son, Wyatt. Three generations of Macys exploring and enjoying the wilds of "the last frontier"!

On July 1, we headed to the Denver airport to catch a flight to Anchorage. On the way, we stopped at the house of Amy's parents, Steve and Sandy Weiner, in Aurora. As we chatted excitedly about the trip, my phone chirped. It was an email from Eco Competitor Relations: "Travis, please give us a call."

Oh, boy. Here we go.

I called.

"So, Trav, do you guys still want to come to Fiji?"

We were in! I thanked the race coordinator and shared the news with Dad and my in-laws. After a round of hoots and hugs, Wyatt, Dad, and I loaded into my truck—Dad's truck—and headed for the airport. My mind was on fire. We were actually going to do it. In the glow of that moment, I had no idea how we would tackle the toughest race in the world, but I knew we would do whatever was required. We would focus on our collective strengths, mitigate weaknesses, lead when we could, and ask for help when we needed it. With a team-oriented ethos, we would move forward doggedly—as fast as we could, as slow as we must.

It was game on for Fiji. The Unknown was out there waiting. And the Macys were coming for it.

SIX

What about "The Guys"?

Wyatt and Gracie and Jaxon are very intelligent kids and sometime, in fact in a very short period of time, they are going to realize I have a very serious illness and, in fact, am going to die. I don't know when that will be, but that's certainly going to be a sad time for all of us.

—*MACE'S JOURNAL*

THE FORTY-NINTH STATE began speaking to me early in my life. I wasn't ready as a child for James Michener's 868-page epic novel *Alaska*, about the fauna, flora, terra firma, seas, sky, and people of the "last frontier" (though I frequently recommend it now), but I was totally game for watching for the millionth time Iditarod dogsled race highlights with Dad on VHS, or hearing his stories about getting lost during— and then winning—the 100-mile Idatashoe snowshoeing race. My previous trips to Alaska with the family had laid the foundation for leading outdoor trips (hiking, backpacking, sea kayaking, rafting) with Overland Adventures up north in 2004 before my senior year of college at CU-Boulder. Dad and I did a weeklong running/snowshoeing race in Canada's Northwest Territory (not Alaska, and not actually very close to it, but still way the hell up there) in 2008, and the summer of 2018 found me accompanying my friend Greg McHale on mountain goat and mountain caribou hunts in the Yukon for his adventure TV show, *Greg McHale's Wild Yukon*. Simply put, Dad and I can't get enough of the far north, and we were totally pumped to get up there with Wyatt, then eight, in July 2019, two months before Eco-Challenge Fiji.

Nothing forces an emphasis on living in the present and creating memories like looming mortality. I knew our seventeen-day odyssey was something special, and I made a point of keeping a daily video journal. Excerpts tell the story of three generations having fun together: an energetic kid who can't get enough of the fishing or of his grandpa; that grandpa, a little uncertain about the daily schedule or how to work the camper but present and enthusiastic and plenty fit enough to keep up with an eight-year-old kid; and a dad, mostly happy and in the moment but also a little stressed in managing the details of a long trip while simultaneously navigating his own waves of sadness and uncertainty. Maybe sometime I'll turn these home videos into a Warren Miller–style film, probably featuring Dad's favorite, "On the Road Again" (original Willie Nelson version, of course), and a posh Instagram-ish filter to make it look classically Alaskan. The scenes might run something like this:

Seated at the bar in a 50's-style diner in Anchorage: Grandfather, Father, and Son wolf down pancakes while telling the camera how excited they are for the upcoming journey: fishing, camping, travel, guys' stuff.

First fish of the trip: Son casts off the beach along the spit in Homer to pull in a Dolly Varden. Grandfather and Father beam with pride in the three-man/one-fish selfie. Three generations partake in a day of guided halibut fishing way out in the ocean. They all catch their limit and box up pounds of white delight to fly home. On a rocky shoreline, Son and Father fish while Grandfather puts in his running miles; uncertain of navigation on roads and trails, he runs back and forth along the beach for hours.

Denali National Park: Father records surreptitiously as the three hike and Grandfather tells Son about the time he trekked through the jungle during the Eco-Challenge in Borneo. We don't see the tears shed by Father—tears of happiness that this is happening and sadness that it might not happen again. Still in Denali, the three get off the bus in the middle of nowhere. Leaving the road, they hike a vast drainage for most of the day through prime grizzly country. Son feels safe because his dad is there. How Father feels, too.

Talkeetna: Northern Exposure—burgers, beer, camping, fishing. At the campground, Father and Son fish while Grandfather snoozes in the camper... but he becomes uncertain of time and, worried that they've been gone too long, runs downriver looking for them. Father finds him wandering around, finally. Little scare but all is well. That's what I told myself.

Fourth of July parade, Soldotna: Candy, flags, fun... our last like this? Sun at midnight (girls in bikinis on top of the RV next to us, Son not quite old enough to appreciate). All three are out playing in the campground, Grandfather with a hilarious impersonation of the day's fishing guide, who kept trying to teach him an intricate casting technique with little regard for the challenges of Alzheimer's. Lots of tangled lines there (and not for the youngest). Back in the camper, all three have underwear on their heads because Son thinks it's so funny! Dad and Grandpa do, too.

Father out running from sea to peak, climbing thousands of feet, bear spray at the ready. Thick fire smoke and glaciers over there (smaller than last time). Global warming? Yup—cognition is not the only thing going to shit. Video entry: tears mix with pride, excitement, and newfound confidence through time together in the outdoors. That could be a good version of the new normal.

Back in Anchorage: same diner, same pancakes. They tell the camera what they each loved best about the trip, and it was the same thing for everyone: fathers and sons.

I tell my kids to avoid the word "awesome" because it usually doesn't really mean anything. But our Alaska trip really did inspire awe, so we'll call it like it was: awesome. Coming back to reality was tough—work, school starting, doctor visits, financial planning for hypotheticals—but that stress was dampened by a new hyperfocus: get ready for Fiji!

My daughter, Lila, loves to sprint across the lawn toward me singing, "Teamwork makes the…" and as she jumps into my arms and we spin—"*dream work*!" We giggle together and smile. Lila may be only eight, but she's right: teamwork really does make the dream work. The team game took effect, full-on, as Eco training peaked that summer. With Shane in Durango, Colorado, and Nellie in Moab, Utah, they'd be doing most of their physical training alone and emailing with me about gear, certifications, plane tickets, and other minutiae. That left Dad and me to train together in Evergreen, often accompanied by Marsh, Dr. Bob, and my good friend Andrew Speers.

A longtime teacher and mountain biking coach at Evergreen High School, Andrew and I met in 2009 when I took an English teaching position at EHS, and we quickly forged a strong friendship through our shared interests in mountain biking, adventure racing, and hunting. When I asked Andrew if he would like to serve as our Team Assistance Crew (TAC) for Fiji, his response was simple: "Uh, you want me to come along for a free adventure trip in Fiji? Lemme think about that... heck, yeah!" Andrew did wait for permission from the school principal before committing for sure, and it was great to know our TAC was just as excited about the event as we were. A salt-of-the-earth Oklahoma boy who can ride a bike, read a map, fix anything, solve problems, and hold his liquor (or, as we found later in the Fijian villages, kava), Andrew is just the kind of guy you want in your camp out in the jungle in the middle of the night. On the racecourse Andrew would be an asset not only to us but to other teams as he chipped in to fix their bikes and crew vehicles, but for now in Evergreen we had him to ourselves. And thankfully, Andrew is an expert in one discipline that would require more practice than usual this time around: the ropes.

In most adventure races, teams encounter fixed-ropes segments that utilize a range of skills and gear. Ropes experts—usually climbing guides, and there were dozens of them from around the world at the Fiji race—set the ropes before the race. The stage is typically some incredible rock crag or canyon or waterfall or alpine peak, the kind of place a climber or mountaineer would drool over. When teams arrive, they navigate the ropes in a predetermined order. Skills utilized typically include traversing a fixed line that's attached to many anchors; ascending a steep, vertical, or overhanging rope using jumars; crossing a Tyrolean traverse, which is a rope strung over a canyon or other gap; and rappelling back down to the ground, often concluded by a dangling drop into water for a swim. The gear is complicated and the skills are dynamic. We've done it during the day, in the middle of the night, in deserts, and over glaciers, and I love it!

Having completed challenging climbs like the Diamond on Longs Peak, Dad was a serious climber in the 1980s, and he typically also loved the ropes in adventure races, often providing the safety oversight and steady hand to guide his teammates and anyone else around who might be shaking in their running shoes. But things had changed with Alzheimer's. Dad had put on a climbing harness literally thousands of times, often in the wet, cold, dark while sleep deprived. Ten years ago he could have done it with his eyes closed and then taught a child to belay. Visual-spatial challenges hit hard though, and now Dad was concerned about the ropes. My friend Jesse from CAMP-USA hooked us up with some top-of-the-line harnesses, gloves, ascenders, carabiners, and slings, and I showed Mom and Dad how the setup worked. After a quick review, Dad could put the harness on correctly and manipulate the twist-lock mechanism on the carabiners.

But the next day, it was all gone: the once-familiar gear now looked and felt like a tangle of random webbing. Sensing no difference between a leg loop and a belay loop, Dad would encounter frustration. "Dang it, Pammy, I swear I had this dialed yesterday! What the hell is going on?!" Dad was fired up. I bet you would be too if you could see relatively simple, ingrained skills disappearing before your eyes.

As always, Mom remained calm and helpful: "Let's take a look at that together, Mace." She'd walk over, put a hand on his arm, help him straighten out the harness, and slowly put it on (leg loops first, one foot, the other, pull up the waist strap, tighten it up). And there they'd remain, as a team, literally for over an hour almost every day, taking a climbing harness off and putting it on again, until Dad was confident he had it dialed. Sometimes my kids would join in, patiently helping Grandpa in and out of harness over and over again until he could do it alone.

And the next day the skill would be gone.

So they'd do it again.

Dad's tenacious work ethic kicked into overdrive. His Eco-Challenge mission was clear, and he biked and ran every day, often with Marsh and sometimes with me, though my schedule of parenting, work, soccer, and gymnastics didn't seem quite as simple as Dad's. After running and biking, Dad would go through his climbing harness routine and then hit the pool or paddle or do some yoga—or all of them.

I also began to appreciate one ironically beautiful aspect of the Alzheimer's journey: the present. When your sense of time is blurred and it's hard to remember what you did yesterday or what's coming tomorrow, all you have is the here and now. Dad was embracing that—he still is—and who was I to worry anxiously about what *might* happen in the jungle in Fiji when I had an incredible opportunity to train with Dad, doing what we love on foot and on the bike in the Colorado Rockies? Right here. Right now.

That dance between full-on, 100 percent commitment to the present moment with a strengths-based focus on the one hand and, on the other, a bit of an eye toward what could be coming down the road became the rhythm of our team's Alzheimer's journey. "To hell with getting affairs in order" really was how we saw it, but we did nonetheless cross the Ts on powers of attorney, a family trust, wills, and finances. "Nothing is going to stop us until the finish line in Fiji" really was what we believed, but I did simultaneously take many steps to manage risk and accept responsibility for pulling the plug on our race, should anything become truly dangerous before or during the event. I used to think life was pretty straightforward: this is good, that's bad, be nice, work hard, things will work out. I still believe that, but now, nearing forty and having faced adversity, I understand the world as less black/white and more gray. And it's also more colorful, sometimes with challenge and despair but also with deeper satisfaction and appreciation. Family grooves at the center of this rich dance floor of life, and in the summer of 2019 I was pumped to be going for something big with my dad.

"*Splash*!" Speaking of big (and cold!), the waves of Clear Creek near Idaho Springs, Colorado, were soon hammering us in the face as we navigated a raft down the fast, narrow river. Dr. Bob had flown out to meet Marsh, Dad, and me for a swiftwater skills certification course with Brett Hochmuth, a local guide based in Evergreen. Swiftwater was just one of the many certifications needed for Eco-Challenge; we'd also be working on fixed-ropes skills and safety, jungle navigation/survival, and first aid.

Brett's course began with some "classroom" instruction delivered outside with a whiteboard at a picnic area near the river. His captivating review of fluid dynamics piqued my interest; we learned that a swimmer usually floats downriver faster than the raft itself because the swimmer's body is in the faster-moving water below the surface. If someone falls out, better get 'em back quick! I was taking notes, and I could tell Dad was also paying close attention, but my eyes watered thinking that, no matter how engaged and attentive he was now, Dad's new learning here might not be accessible tomorrow. As with many of the skills for Eco, we'd probably be relying more on Dad's decades of experience—and hopefully the innate movements and intuitions therein—than on anything new. For the whitewater, we'd also be relying heavily on Shane, who spent years as a rafting guide and competed internationally for Team USA in the two-man slalom canoe.

Back at the training course, Dr. Bob and I took turns

steering the raft through fast rapids while Dad and Marsh paddled. Bob and I were both good enough with the ruddering and J-strokes, and we made it through some tight spots without flipping or getting stuck. We practiced safe whitewater swimming technique—butt down, feet forward—and tossed throw bags to each other, practicing rescue techniques that might be needed in Fiji. Training in demanding conditions is often helpful, and this Colorado snowmelt was definitely colder and probably faster than what we'd see in Fiji!

Prerace newsletters indicated the possibility of trekking and carrying bikes across multiple fast-moving rivers, and Brett spent about an hour working us through a range of strategies for that. When crossing a fast river—and usually the rocks in fast rivers are *slippery*—you typically want to connect with teammates for added stability. A larger and/or more stable person will be positioned upstream to block some of the current, and you might even use a pole or stick for added stability. A collegiate football player (way back when, but he's still a beast), Dr. Bob was our blocker. He took most of the current while Marsh, Dad, and I held close, navigating the current and rocks by feel. Dad's balance was surprisingly good, and the experience bolstered my confidence as I looked ahead to Fiji, where we'd surely cross dozens of streams and rivers by foot and with bikes. Brett felt good about our performance as a group and individually, and he enthusiastically signed off on our certifications.

Next up was ropes training. Jesse connected us with an experienced rock climbing guide who'd set up fixed ropes and assess our readiness according to Eco's certification process. Dad continued to prepare for this day, and we all approached the trial with some anxiety and uncertainty: How would the ropes skills test go? And what if Alzheimer's made some of the skills impossible?

A hot summer morning at North Table Mountain in

Golden, Colorado, found Dr. Bob, Marsh, Dad, and me hiking a rocky trail up to a popular sport-climbing crag. Amy and I lived at the base of this hill just after college, and I knew the place was crawling—or maybe slithering—with rattlesnakes. We met the guide at the cliffs, and he had already set an impressive and complicated ropes circuit involving a technical traverse with multiple anchors along a handline; a challenging ascent up a vertical and overhanging rope; a long Tyrolean traverse across a fifty-foot canyon; and a nice rappel back to the start (simple, other than the possibility of putting your foot on a sunbathing rattler). No need to understand all of these terms; in a nutshell, we'd be scrambling all over rocky cliffs, constantly clipping and unclipping carabiners and other gear, utilizing a wide range of skills. Again, these are all things Dad had done for decades, and he previously would have been the leader for Team Stray Dogs in this sort of scenario.

We were all using brand-new gear from CAMP-USA. It was the best stuff made, but we knew some adjustments for sling lengths and relative positions would be needed. Dr. Bob drew the short straw and tackled the circuit first. He nailed it... until the Tyrolean traverse. Imagine dangling from a line strung over a canyon. If the rope breaks, you fall about seventy-five feet onto hard rock—but it looks a whole lot higher because you're way up on a cliff that's way up on a mountain. You can see the Coors Brewery down below (yup, it really is "somewhere near Golden, Colorado," but it's not nearly as snowy as the commercials), and a cold one is probably all you want right now, especially since this whole thing is happening about 5,000 feet higher than the place you live. And then your phone slides out of your pocket, smashing and bouncing down the mountain before you spend the next twenty minutes doing awkward pull-ups on the line, trying to get yourself to the other side.

That was Dr. Bob. And he smiled the whole way through.

Turns out the sling connecting Dr. Bob's harness to the fixed Tyrolean line was too long, and that's why it was so tough to get across. Everyone else's was too long as well, but after watching Bob the adjustment was simple, and Marsh and I cruised through the circuit. Dad was next, and we were all nervous. This is what Dad had spent so many hours preparing for. He'd put in more total training time (and WAY more ropes time) than any of us, and his fitness was high. Heck, I knew Dad could outrun most of my thirty- and forty-something endurance clients in a running race up Evergreen Mountain.

But this wasn't a running race up Evergreen Mountain. Although things were smooth for Dad after I helped him clip in for a rappel or an ascent, managing multiple slings and clipping and reclipping the carabiners for a multiple-anchored fixed line proved just beyond reach that day. The visual-spatial limitations made it impossible for him to tell which rope was which as he passed fixed anchors on a line. We all had a blast and the guide did a great job composing a very professional, thorough assessment of Dad's current capabilities for the certification process. Simply put, it was clear that, due to the limitations from Alzheimer's, Dad would need some support on the ropes in Fiji from his teammates and/or the climbing guides onsite.

These arduous events tend to foster a family atmosphere between competitors and organizers, and that's very true for Eco-Challenge. Producer Lisa Hennessy and race director Kevin Hodder were particularly supportive in getting Dad to the race. Kev and I talked at length about potential safety concerns regarding fixed ropes, and we agreed on a plan to support Dad on those parts of the course. Eco always hires some of the world's top climbing guides to set and monitor the ropes. We agreed that safety and fairness could be achieved through a bit of extra support from a climbing guide who might travel next to Dad and make sure all carabiners were clipped and unclipped correctly.

Anyone who's ever gone mountain biking, backpacking, rafting, rock climbing, and/or camping knows each of those activities requires extensive gear. Well, imagine gathering all of that stuff at once—plus a week's worth of food and medical supplies for just about any scenario up to and including the jungle virus, leptospirosis—and bringing it with you to Fiji. Needless to say, gear prep and management presented a significant challenge before and during the Eco-Challenge.

The mandatory gear list covered fourteen pages and included: shell jacket, fleece top, emergency waterproof strobe lamp, headlamp, signal mirror, survival blanket, compass, lighter or matches, knife, whistle, emergency smoke canister, first aid kit (consisting of twelve specific items), radio, race passport, duct tape, emergency GPS tracker, altimeter watch, race maps, tarp, waterproof map bags, machete, bivvy sack, shovel (for digging a hole to poop in), paracord, waterproof duffel bag, five forty-eight-gallon gear boxes, four bike boxes, tent, sleeping bags, sleeping pads, camping chairs, mountain bikes, bike helmets, flashing lights for bikes, bike repair kit, climbing harness, climbing helmet, climbing gloves, rappel device, hollow block, ascenders, lanyards, foot loops, carabiners, personal flotation device (life jacket), river knife, throw bag, outrigger canoe paddles, dive mask, underwater light, glow sticks, emergency flares, bailing bucket, and righting line.

Looking back more than twenty years, I remember Dad gathering and packing all of his gear for the early Eco-Challenges. He'd be up late using AOL on our dial-up Internet connection to communicate with sponsors, and then opening boxes of bars and clothing and shoes, and then putting every-thing in well-organized piles as the race drew closer. His attention to detail was paramount: calories counted, stuff sacks labeled, all contingencies considered. As a kid, I thought all the gear was super cool, and I remember sifting through the piles, admiring the new ice ax or climbing helmet, and asking Dad if I could have—or just borrow—those sweet sunglasses or the rain jacket. He of course needed most of the items for his races, but he often made me feel special by lending or giving some item here or there—with a caveat: "Someday, Bud, you're going to be the sponsored athlete, and I sure hope you remember to take care of your dad when that time comes."

Well, with Fiji approaching, "someday" had arrived, full-on. For years I had been hooking Dad up with shoes, hats, and clothing from my sponsors (most of whom were generally excited to have him wearing their stuff as well), but this was the first time I had been managing all of the gear for a race we'd be doing together. Given the impacts of Alzheimer's—so much for attention to detail and counting calories for food bags—I harbored no hard feelings about taking over for Dad on the gear front, but it was definitely a lot of work. Daily emails with Shane and Nellie kept us on the same page: we had three carbon canoe paddles but needed a fourth; Shane still had his machete from Fiji 2002 and would sharpen it; some climbing equipment had changed and we'd need to practice the hollow block (a pre-tied rope device designed to keep climbers safe while rappelling); yes, my mother-in-law, Sandy, had volunteered to sew six required patches onto four race jerseys apiece for us; Evergreen Bicycle Outfitters would hook us up with a great price on Cannondale bikes; and on and on. Dad was putting in the training, and I was wading through gear in my basement. The stress was high at times (and so were the credit card bills!), but I had to smile when my own kids showed interest in my piles of stuff, often helping me organize Grandpa's items—and asking to borrow things for their own adventures.

I simultaneously engaged in contingency planning as never before. Shane, Nellie, and I had not competed in a big, international adventure race like this since prior to having children of our own. Back at that time (the 2000s) we were racing together and against each other on top teams, going for the podium and sometimes taking—at least in hindsight— questionable risks to go for speed, prize money, sponsorship, and glory. I was pleased that we could all agree early in planning for this event that coming home to our kids was paramount. And getting Dad home to his grandkids is where the contingency planning came in.

"So, Doc, what do you think about the possible risks of Dad doing the Eco-Challenge?"

"Well, there's not exactly a precedent for people with Alzheimer's doing long adventure races in the jungle."

"Well... "

"I can tell you that sometimes cognitive decline accelerates rapidly when the patient experiences infection. Sleep deprivation would almost definitely not be good. You know about the injury and overuse risks better than I do. All of that said, I can absolutely see why you guys would want to do something big and special like this."

I'm paraphrasing here, but Dad, Mom, and I really did hold such a conversation with his doctor, who generally was supportive and encouraging of our belief that, while Eco-Challenge certainly carried some risk, there was also a possibly greater risk of throwing in the towel, staying home, and calling it all good on a life lived fully.

The doctor had made great points about infection and sleep deprivation. We knew most teams would be sleeping very little, as we had in the past; a common strategy was to race through the first night and then sleep for one to two hours the following nights. That surely wouldn't work with Alzheimer's. Not sleeping much also leads to saturated feet because they never dry out. The skin becomes puffed, cracked, flaky, and painful; sometimes trench foot develops. I had learned that leptospirosis, a nasty jungle bug common to Fiji's freshwaters, could enter the body not only through drinking and cuts but also via saturated—and apparently permeable—skin on the feet.

I knew we'd need to lead the race in time spent sleeping. To prepare for that, we ordered bigger packs from OutThere USA (owned by Mike Kloser, another old friend of Dad's who'd be racing as well) and planned to carry more gear than usual: a tiny cookstove and pot to make hot meals at night and coffee in the morning; inflatable sleeping pads that were big enough to provide actual comfort; extra socks; Dad's supplements and probiotics to hopefully keep nastiness at bay; hardy emergency bivvy bags to sleep in each night. Thankfully, nightly sleep would also help greatly with the foot issues because they could dry sufficiently while we slumbered. Knowing the increased risk of falls in steep terrain and scrambles due to visual-spatial challenges and loss of balance, I worked closely with Jesse to practice a variety of belay techniques that would potentially allow me to scramble up or down a pitch, rig an anchor (likely from a tree), and then belay Dad so he could safely ascend or descend. To clarify, we knew the fixed ropes set by Eco-Challenge staff would be bullet-proof; the uncertainty lay in technical terrain (sans fixed ropes but still steep and dangerous) that we might experience while trekking, biking, or canyoneering.

Finally, on September 4, 2019, my truck (Dad's truck) was totally loaded for our journey to Denver International Airport. It's a good thing we had a big truck because the load was massive: three forty-eight-gallon gear boxes, two bike boxes, a snowboard bag carrying a bunch of paddles (and other items to get it right up to the fifty pounds allowed by airlines), a few duffels, and one racing pack each as a carry-on item (also loaded to fifty pounds). Mom snapped a photo of Dad, Andrew, and me in the parking lot at Evergreen High School (a herd of elk down on the soccer field, as usual), and we hit the road.

I've gotten the feeling over the years that airports and their staff don't like adventure racers. And who can blame them? We show up with a whole bunch of big, heavy, dirty stuff. Half of it looks like bombs, and we have plenty of ziplock baggies full of white powder. We're usually in a rush, and our itineraries are highly complicated.

The check-in attendants can see us coming rows away, and I have learned to scope them out as I make my way through the line. Hassled person? Pass. Detail-oriented curmudgeon who probably reads the guidelines every day? No way. Smiley newbie who might not know about all possible charges and is probably excited to hear about our fun trip to Fiji? Now that's my checker! Somehow I made it to her desk, and things worked out so well that Andrew and I were soon repacking some of the gear boxes—yup, full-on gear explosion, right there in the busy DIA lines, and not for the first time—because, somehow, there would be *no overweight charges* this time and we could save hundreds of dollars by consolidating gear. It was a small win, but I know from experience that small victories add up to big progress, and things seemed to be shaping up nicely as we headed overseas.

SEVEN

*Almost every day someone asks me how I'm doing,
and I reply, "Pretty good for an old guy," and
sometimes add, "...an old guy with Alzheimer's,"
if the person I'm talking to is aware of it. And
it's true. I usually am pretty darn good. And the
reason I say that is because people don't really
want to hear about my troubles or anyone else's.*

*But today I just woke up angry. To be honest,
there are days like today that I am just goddamn
angry that I have this disease and there's nothing
I can do about it. I have always been a happy
person, but this disease seems to be testing me.*

*Obviously, I can't let this disease change my
normal good nature and relationships with my
friends and family. ALZ may just be a test to see how
much I can take. Getting mad doesn't help, but it
seems, at least for the time being, ALZ always wins.*

I will do anything possible to win the test.

—MACE'S JOURNAL

I AWOKE TO THE WHITE HUM of a jet plane cruising across
the South Pacific. Outside the window of the Airbus 330, the
Melanesian skies were tranquil.

But Dad wasn't.

"Damn it," he was muttering, as he fidgeted in the seat,
poking the video screen on the seat-back facing him with his
index finger, again and again. "How the hell...?"

"Dad," I murmured. "What's the matter?"

"Oh, sorry to wake you, Bud," he said. "It's this goddamn TV. Everybody else is watching movies and I can't even get 'em to start playing."

I looked over. This wasn't a touch screen. "You need to use this, Dad," I said, helping him lift the remote control out of its holster by his elbow.

In fairness to Dad, these onboard entertainment systems aren't always the most intuitive technology. But Dad had already battled with the seatbelt when we boarded at LAX—when was it? Ten hours ago? "I've never seen one like this," he had grumbled when we sat down. It was a standard airline seatbelt, the type he had successfully buckled and unbuckled a thousand times before in his well-traveled life.

By now, eleven months after his diagnosis of early-onset Alzheimer's, I was getting used to his fresh moments of confusion, when he'd draw a blank on how to put on a shirt or hold a toothbrush.

I just hoped those moments wouldn't get us into serious trouble in the jungle.

We were beginning our descent into Nadi, the third largest city and the transportation hub of the Republic of Fiji. The 2019 Eco-Challenge would be starting in three days. Not for the first or last time, I found myself wondering:

Was this really a good idea? Was dragging my dad to the other side of the world and plopping him in the middle of a Fijian rain forest really the right thing to do?

This is 400 miles of strange surroundings and difficult conditions. It would be disorienting enough to anyone, much less a man with a degenerative brain disease. What the hell was I thinking when I even suggested this?

The abrupt strike of wheels on tarmac and an announcement over the PA system interrupted my doubting inner voice.

"Welcome to Nadi Airport," said the honey-voiced flight attendant. "We hope you have enjoyed your flight on Fiji Airways. *Bula!*"

"Bula!" responded a ragged chorus of jet-lagged passengers, many of them, like us, traveling to Fiji for the race.

This term, I'd learned, is equivalent to *aloha* in Hawaii: While it commonly translates to "welcome," bula is an all-purpose word; it's often used to describe the warm and generous spirit of the people who live on this cluster of volcanic islands 2,765 miles southwest of Honolulu. As a Lonely Planet guidebook describes it, Fiji is a "hallucination of paradise," with its turquoise waters, lush jungles, and white, secluded beaches.

The bula spirit is no illusion, though. The indigenous people here are Polynesian, although there is a large Indian population as well. Regardless of the ethnicity, the Fijians we met over the next three weeks were unfailingly warm, polite, and hospitable, even when confronted with a bunch of cranky, sleep-deprived Americans filing off a plane.

Patience is part of the job description for any parent and educator, and I pride myself on having a fairly deep reservoir of that essential ingredient. But even my forbearance was tested by a passport-control process that seemed to go on for hours. Keeping up that bula spirit apparently means keeping out microbes and pathogens that could infect this remote Eden, as every one of us, from hairline to shoe sole, was carefully checked to make sure we weren't inadvertently bringing in some contagion (and this was months before the COVID-19 pandemic).

Then there was baggage pickup. Think about the last time you claimed luggage at an airport. A circle of passengers forms around the conveyor belt; a klaxon blares as the belt noisily grinds into action and begins disgorging suitcases from its maw. One by one, those waiting pick out their bag, maybe two. In the rare case of a large family, someone might have a trolley on hand to pack up several.

Baggage claim for a group of adventure racers is more like the arrival of supplies to a besieged city. It's chaos: The belts and luggage carts in Nadi groaned with mountain bikes, backpacks that appeared ready to sustain an assault on Everest, huge seventy-pound Rubbermaid shipping containers packed with the items included on the official fourteen-page Eco-Challenge Mandatory Gear List— accessories large and small that included everything from climbing harnesses to magnetic compasses, water purification tablets to paddleboard repair kits. Team members wait, jostling to get their stuff, carefully hoisting container-ship–sized boxes off a moving belt.

None of this fazed Dad in the least. He could get rattled by a seat belt but he remained poised, even cheerful, amidst the glacially paced checkpoint lines and suitcase pandemonium.

"You know, Trav, if there's one thing I'm good at," he reminded me, "it's waiting around."

Admittedly, that is an overlooked secret to success in endurance racing. Even runners who've done more conventional races, such as the New York City and Boston Marathons, will tell you that. Because of security, road closures and other logistics, you typically have to get to the staging area hours and hours before these races start. What do you do for that time? You wait. Those who can do it without expending valuable energy fretting about the pain and discomfort they're about to subject themselves to are usually the more successful racers.

This waiting-around factor is even greater in our rarefied world of ultradistance and adventure racing, because while there are fewer competitors, there's usually more stuff involved and in less accessible places. I recalled scenes in some of the early Eco-Challenge competitions Dad had done and that I had watched on YouTube in the months leading up to our race: Teams would be lined up for hours in some remote corner of the globe, waiting to swim across the freezing rapids of a river, or rappel down a jagged cliff over an abyss. And again—unlike, say, the New York City Marathon—there's no thirteen-lane Verrazzano Bridge for everyone to spread out on, just a narrow, muddy trail where competitors stand until it's their turn to suffer.

So, waiting is part of the game. Even waiting for our gear in Nadi International Airport.

Amidst all this pent-up energy and confusion, Dad was in his element. He'll chat with anybody, especially a captive audience of first-time adventure racers—including the team of buff, twenty-something Crossfitters from Los Angeles. With his lean frame and gray beard, he had the look of a sagacious veteran, and I noticed them listening intently as Dad declaimed about races past, including some crazy thing that happened to him and his teammate Marshall Ulrich in Borneo in the 2000 Eco-Challenge. I'd heard this one before—something to do with running through a cave covered ankle-deep in bat guano.

"You believe that shit?" Dad said, chuckling, as he concluded his tale. "I can't believe we had to do that."

I noticed eyes widen among the studly competitors from LA. While I'm sure some of them thought Dad was bat-shit crazy, I half expected others in earshot to turn around and head back to the plane after hearing such war stories. Dad didn't want to scare anybody, however. On the contrary: Racing and this race in particular were woven into the fabric of his soul. He wanted to share it with the world, and he was always encouraging to those who were going to accept the challenge. "Don't worry," I heard him say several times to different people during the long morning of processing and baggage pickup. "Just take care of each other out there and you'll have the greatest experience of your life. Hey, it's the Eco-Challenge!"

The Eco-Challenge. The World's Toughest Race, as it was now being advertised. In its televised form, it had begun with an abridged forty-five-minute highlight reel shown on MTV as part of the X-Games in 1995. In 1996 it was aired as a three-part documentary on the Discovery Channel, a broadcast that won Mark Burnett his first Emmy. Seventy teams competed in that race, and only thirteen finished the 400-mile trek through the wilds of British Columbia.

One of the teams that year was the Stray Dogs, led by two Colorado ultramarathoners, Marshall and my dad.

I had watched that first Discovery Channel Eco-Challenge in the months leading up to Fiji. Aside from the amusing preponderance of 1990s short shorts, mullets, mustaches, and garish Oakley eyewear (all of which are again popular with Millennials), it was notable for the visual and emotional power of the story, and for delving into the motivations of those who had left modern comforts for the remote rapids and cliffs of western Canada.

Watching it now, it's easy to see how Burnett reimagined the Eco-Challenge as a reality drama. Many of the same elements that would make *Survivor* such a phenomenon a few years later are here in the 1996 Discovery Channel broadcast: the long, lingering shots of an imposing, exotic landscape; the haunting, ethereal music; the reverential bows to indigenous culture; and, of course, the personal and team odysseys that are really at the heart of the story.

"Epic," recalled Burnett in a 2011 interview, when asked about the challenges of organizing the first editions of the Eco-Challenge. "It was really like a military operation."

As a competitor rewatching this classic broadcast, I was eager to see more of adventure race legends like New Zealand's John Howard and Ian Adamson, whose Team Eco-Internet won that 1996 competition in British Columbia. But it was the human-interest stories that took center stage in the broadcast, the normal-looking individuals testing themselves in these outlandish, harrowing situations: a seventy-three-year-old grandmother trying to navigate a Tyrolean rope climb; an attractive Houston attorney who applied lipstick before each event nearly drowning in a frigid river; a team of suburban weekend warriors wildly out of their depth but desperately trying to make the checkpoints as they faded farther and farther behind.

Viewers got to watch teams frayed at the nerves, coming apart due to lack of sleep, the terrain, the effort, or the sheer audacity of what they were attempting to do. But there was also caring and love and acts of cooperation: the racer who proposed to the team's crew member at the finish line; the impromptu merger between the French and American teams that had competed for second place through most of the race and who—as their injuries mounted and the race took its toll—decided to create a détente, join forces, and finish the race as one combined unit of new comrades.

All of that was in the 1996 broadcast. And now, *we* were going to be part of the show, nearly twenty-five years later. Burnett and his coproducer Lisa Hennessy were in the business of finding compelling story angles from the participants. They respected us as serious competitors, but they didn't pick Team Endure for the 2020 reboot because it was good old, affable Mace who had competed in all eight editions of the original Eco-Challenge and could tell funny stories about running through bat shit.

They knew what was compelling here: A veteran and likable competitor now battling Alzheimer's disease as well as the jungle? His team, led by his son, trying to get him through this race, despite that? Not to mention the presence of our teammate Danelle, who had survived a near-death experience in an earlier Eco-Challenge and was now back in a selfless effort to assist her friend Mace?

Check.

Check.

Check.

Yup, all the ingredients for heart-tugging reality TV: likable characters, exotic terrain, serious illness.

But what might make for compelling reality viewing to an audience watching the show on Amazon Prime in the summer of 2020 was about to become reality for me here in Fiji in September 2019. Dad couldn't even figure out how to buckle a seat belt on a plane. And it was going to be my responsibility to get this man through the most grueling endurance challenge on the planet and bring him back home safe and sound.

"Trav, could you give me a hand with this?" called Shane, as our gear came rolling around the baggage-claim belt.

Again, I tried to banish the doubts and get focused.

We had a race to run.

Fortified a bit by a cup of espresso I'd found at a coffee bar in the airport, I emerged from our stuffed-to-the-gills airport van to a scene of splendor: the Pullman Nadi Bay Resort and

Spa, the five-star hotel that would be our home for two days before the race start. This was Eco-Challenge headquarters. Flags with the race logo flew proudly (if a bit languidly in the tropical humidity) by the grand entrance. Competitors, crew, and hotel staff scurried about. The five of us—my dad and I, Shane, Danelle, and Andrew—were ushered to a check-in area, where I met many of the race staff I'd been corresponding with for months by email.

There was show-runner Lisa Hennessy, walking by with a cell phone in her hand, surrounded by an entourage of staff members. Like many of those on the current production team, she remembered my dad from the old days and had encouraged our participation in the race. "You made it!" she said as she bustled down the corridor. "Great to see you guys."

"Hey, Lisa, nice to see you too," replied Dad.

It occurred to me that my dad probably hadn't seen her in over a decade—I'd been the one in touch with Lisa during the planning for this year's race. Yet he recognized her and recalled her name instantly. The same man who couldn't remember how to unlock the front door of his house.

Not for the first time, I thought, what a strange disease Alzheimer's is.

At the check-in area in the lobby we also saw Kevin Hodder, the technical race director. While it would be presented like a TV show, the Eco-Challenge is not a scripted event; a real race was about to take place, and Kevin was the man who had to make sure it would come off. Originally a ski guide from British Columbia, he had been part of the crew for the 1996 Eco-Challenge and had worked his way up the ranks of Burnett's organization. He was now well known and respected in the adventure racing world. It was Hodder who, along with his colleague Scott Flavelle, had actually scouted out the entire 400-mile course of our race, a route that would be kept secret until the morning of the race, forcing us competitors to start navigating on the fly. At this point we had a vague idea of what we'd be doing: trekking, climbing, paddling, traversing, mountain biking are typical Eco-Challenge disciplines. But how long, how high, how deep, under exactly what conditions—we could only guess.

Kevin had told me on a phone call a few months earlier that he had confidence in my judgment during the race. Meaning, essentially, that he was relying on me to make tough decisions along the way.

The Eco-Challenge requires improvisation on the part of each team. That's part of what makes it such riveting television. It could mean, for example, pausing for hours to wait for daylight before attempting a technical section on a climb or traverse; opting for a risky shortcut at a critical point in the race; or even deciding that a team had gone as far as it could go. While every team in the Fiji race would have to make decisions along the way and deal with injuries—sprains, fractures, bites, and bruises, not to mention the sheer exhaustion that would beset many—none of them except ours would need to factor Alzheimer's disease into the equation. If it got to a point where continuing the race might put Dad at risk, Kevin was counting on me to put ego aside, put safety first—and drop out of the race.

"I know that under normal circumstances, you'd probably be here trying to win this," Kevin said. "But I have to be able to trust you to make the safe call."

"Kevin," I said, embracing some of the nuanced thinking forced upon me by the Alzheimer's journey, "if we have to do it, we'll do it. Don't worry."

While I was prepared to stop if Alzheimer's left us no choice, Kevin also knew that we were coming to Fiji not to earn sympathy votes but to finish. This wasn't going to be some token one-day demonstration in the jungle, followed by a couple weeks of recuperative luxury back at the five-star hotel.

We were ready to push, ready to race, ready to endure. All of us—including and maybe especially Dad.

"I'm not going there so you guys can do all the work," he said. "If I can't be a real part of the team and pull my own weight, then we shouldn't do this."

Dad was serious, and he'd trained hard for this. We'd climbed, we'd paddled, we'd biked, we'd trekked. Physically, outside of some nagging lower-back issues that had flared up, he was in great shape.

But most of our training around Evergreen had been during the day. Some of the best drama in an adventure race takes place in darkness. The top teams sleep very little and often press on through the night to open up a lead or keep from falling behind. But nighttime can be challenging for those with Alzheimer's. So-called "sundowning"—the behavioral problems that begin at dusk and continue through the night—had disoriented my dad some evenings in Evergreen, Colorado. How would it affect him when night descended over the Fijian jungle?

vAlong with waiting around, one thing my dad is good at is talking. That skill would serve us well for the first two days in Fiji. Barely an hour after we'd arrived at the resort, we were ushered over to the press room, where media people from all over the world were engaged in impromptu interviews with the teams. An Australian morning TV show was actually broadcasting live from the lobby. They had a whole set constructed, including a couch for guests. We'd been one of the teams selected to be interviewed by the show's host, who cheerfully asked us questions about where we were from, our goals in the race. She seemed genuinely impressed and moved by what Dad was trying to achieve.

Not all of the media in attendance, however, had bothered to read the background materials.

"So, what makes your team unique?" asked one rumpled reporter, who I noticed was half-looking over my shoulder as he asked the question, probably to see if he could snag Bear Grylls or Mark Burnett for an interview instead.

"Well," I replied, "we have my dad here, and he has Alzheimer's."

"Right," he said, scribbling halfheartedly in his notebook, and then stopped midstroke.

"Wait...did you say Alzheimer's?"

"Yup."

He looked at my dad. "You...you have Alzheimer's?"

"I wish I could say no," Dad said, grinning. "But yes, I do. Early-onset."

I don't know what this guy expected an Alzheimer's patient to look or act like. He seemed shocked that Dad could even form a sentence and that he wasn't drooling.

"Why are you doing this?" he asked, incredulously— and somewhat insensitively, in my opinion.

Dad took no umbrage.

"Well, I've done every Eco-Challenge, and I wanted to do this one with my son," he said, putting his arm around me. "I also want to show people all over the world battling this disease that they can get out, too, and they can still do what's important to them. And that they still have a voice that can be heard."

Dad's voice certainly could be heard that day. Loud and clear.

I don't think I was ever prouder of him.

The thing about this disease is how quickly it turns. The end of a long first day in Fiji found the five of us in our suite at the Pullman. The resort was decorated in a motif that looked vaguely Native American. Mosaic vector patterns—repeating sequences of geometric shapes—decorated the walls and floors.

Dad and I shared a spacious room, which had a sliding door connecting us to the pool area, the perimeter of which was lined with sleek reclining couches and elegant patio umbrellas. The spacious deck was bathed in an artsy array of lights—different colors, shining from different angles—as techno music blared.

To this unusual tableau we added a few touches: gear from Team Endure and others whose rooms fronted the pool soon accumulated around the deck. Bikes, helmets, backpacks, climbing harnesses, and headlamps soon shared space with the Native art.

"Quite a scene," joked Shane, as we prepared to head to our respective rooms for bed.

That night, while I was deep asleep, Dad woke up, saw the strange, flashing lights outside the sliding door, and went outside onto the pool area, which was by then empty. He wandered around, dumbfounded, tiptoeing around the now-unfamiliar racing gear and staring at the mysterious-looking mosaics, as if they were runes in an alien language or messages he couldn't decipher.

He genuinely believed that he had somehow landed in another world.

Or at least that's what he told us over breakfast.

I think the spoonful of yogurt froze halfway into my mouth when I heard this. "Dad," I exclaimed. "You sure this wasn't some crazy dream?"

"Nope," he said. "I woke up and had no idea where I

was. I really thought that I was...I don't know...somewhere else. Another dimension? Abducted by aliens? Who knows? It scared the hell out of me."

Shane, Andrew, and Nellie glanced at me and laughed nervously. "Mace," Shane said. "I don't blame you. Those mosaics and lights are kinda weird."

I wasn't laughing, however. This was unnerving. We hadn't even started the race. Heck, we hadn't even left the race hotel, and my dad was having problems.

The doubting voices returned.

The morning of the race we were at the staging area, near a remote village called Draubuta, located near a river on Viti Levu, Fiji's largest island. Out of the predawn darkness, three shapes appeared.

"Travis?" I heard one say. "Is there a Travis here?"

"That's me," I said. "Good morning."

"You're gonna wear this microphone the whole race," said a young American voice, ignoring any niceties. Before I could say another word, I felt hands on my neck and back as the sound crew fastened a necklace around my throat and attached it to a neoprene belt that I felt them sliding on, like I was a two-year-old being dressed by his parents.

"Don't touch this," barked the lead sound guy. "We'll be out on the course and we'll take it off when we need to swap out the battery."

And just like that they disappeared back into the darkness.

"Weren't they nice?" I asked sarcastically, shaking my head.

"Be careful what you say now, Trav," joked Shane.

"That's the idea. They want me to blurt out whatever comes into my head."

It was another reminder, of course, that the Eco-Challenge was going to be unlike any endurance competition I'd ever done:

This was a race, but it was also a TV show, and we were now cast members.

This was a race, but we weren't really competing to win, just attempting to finish.

This was a race, but our main opponent, besides the Fijian jungle, was the amyloid plaques in Dad's brain.

Nothing I could do about those, I mused glumly, and then banished the thought.

Competition or no, we were looking at 400 miles of... well...something. We still didn't quite know, but we were certain it would begin with us trying to sail a *camakau*—the traditional singled-sailed Fijian water craft that's like an outrigger canoe—for which we had received about three minutes of training the day before.

And before we knew what, we had to know where. One of the many challenges in the Eco-Challenge is that competitors don't get to see the course until just before the start. Again, to compare it to more traditional endurance races, if you run a marathon, you're focused on running, not on figuring out the route. The way ahead is clearly marked with mileage signs or clocks or balloons or, in a trail race, blazes on a tree. And if that's not enough, race staff or volunteers are typically stationed at key crossroads to make sure you don't go off course.

In an adventure race, the only identifiable parts of the course are the start, the finish, and the checkpoints, probably forty or fifty of them scattered along the 400-mile course broken into about twenty segments, through which we would be expected to climb, paddle, traverse, ride, or trek. Going off course is almost expected.

One of the many skills competitors had to master for success in a race like this was navigation. As in, reading a map and plotting your coordinates. Navigation was my job for Team Endure. As a former high school math teacher, I understood the basics of triangulation and I could calculate sums in my head pretty quickly. (I'm sure you've guessed by now that, in keeping with the spirit of the Eco-Challenge, we wouldn't be allowed to carry iPhones or use a GPS or calculator in the jungle.)

It would have been a lot easier if I could have had the map weeks earlier; I could have plotted a nice, precise course for us on my laptop at home in Colorado. But of course, that defeats the purpose of adventure racing. It's supposed to be... well...an adventure, and part of that is the prospect that you might get lost!

And because this was a made-for-television event, not only did we learn the route five minutes before the start; the very unveiling of the course and the distribution of maps to all teams would be done with great dramatic flourish.

There have been some great Eco-Challenge kickoffs in the past: The '96 race is particularly memorable, as it involved teams riding horseback and running for the first forty miles, which made it look like some kind of bizarre cattle drive in the Old West, except with cowboys in neoprene shorts and Nikes, herding runners instead of cows.

Still, I must say, in all the Eco-Challenges I've watched and all of the editions of the race my dad had competed in, there was never a "course reveal" like the one in Fiji.

The competitors—all 280 of us—had walked about a mile from where we'd stayed the night before the race to the banks of a river, where a stage was set up. A producer went over some last-minute instructions, and then in the distance we heard the roar of engines.

"Look!" said Nellie, pointing skyward.

Four helicopters roared overhead at about tree-level height.

Hanging from the side of one of them was Edward Michael "Bear" Grylls.

We'd met Bear at the hotel when we arrived. He was friendly, enthusiastic, and actually seemed to know who we were, no mean feat considering how many competitors were here.

Now he was looking every inch the former Royal Marine commando that he was before becoming a TV star. Tan, athletic build, close-cropped military haircut. He even had his own machete—the letters BG carved on its handle—sticking out of his backpack.

As the other three choppers hovered nearby, his descended to just four feet or so from the ground. Nonchalantly, as if this was his normal daily routine, Bear hopped off the skids, landed easily on the ground, and loped across the field and up onto the stage.

"Now that's an entrance," said Dad, approvingly.

"Are you ready?" Bear called.

"Yeahhhh," was the collective roar in response from the teams, assembled in front of the stage.

We knew what came next: Behind him was the course map, covered by a canvas sheet with the Eco-Challenge logo. Bear ripped off the sheet to reveal a map of Fiji, with a route clearly marked.

"This is your goal!" he said, pointing to a spot on the map that indicated the finish.

As he spoke, race officials were fanning out, distributing the detailed map coordinates to the team captains.

We were ready now to start the race, to board the camakaus that were moored along the shore. Nearby, a line of local villagers stood and applauded.

"Bula! Bula!" they cried, high-fiving us as we walked toward the shore.

"Bula, Bud!" my dad said, pounding me affectionately on the shoulder. "It's the Eco-Challenge! We made it!"

Yes, I thought. We made it—to the start, at least. As to what wild place we were headed, however, I wasn't quite sure.

EIGHT

Becoming a Legend

Over the years, as I entered my later fifties and sixties, I have become a "legend" in the ultra-distance and worldwide adventure races. The truth is, it's pretty easy to become a legend in this world of sport, if you are around long enough and race enough. In fact, if the truth be known, I'm not particularly good at anything, but I can suffer as well as anyone and simply not quit.

—MACE'S JOURNAL

"THREE...TWO...ONE...GO!"

Bear's countdown sent the race off. Cameras rolled as helicopters hovered, pushing down the jungle foliage like a scene from a Vietnam movie. The locals cheered enthusiastically: "*Bula, bula, bula!*" Racers launched themselves from the bank to their camakaus, eager to finally start the odyssey for which they'd waited so long. Only about ten teams had a real shot at winning this thing—and all of them knew that being in the lead around the first bend meant absolutely nothing in a weeklong race. I constantly tell my coaching clients that most athletes in most long races start too fast, and that's just what happened here. Most teams dug in, paddling hard like it was a 100-meter dash and yelling like it was a floating rodeo.

And when the boats started crashing into each other and tipping over, the scene actually looked a bit like a rodeo! I know, because I watched it from the shore. As the top Kiwi team capsized when a less-experienced team hit them and a competitive Australian team limped to shore with a hole in the boat after being pronged by another craft, we patiently sat on the shore, finishing our maps before pushing off.

Walking to the boats before the race, Shane's experience was evident: "Shit, guys. These boats are really crowded here, and there's going to be chaos at the start." We knew he was right. Carnage-filled starting-line scenes were a hallmark of Burnett's Eco-Challenge footage: horses bucking in Patagonia, camels sprinting in Morocco, homemade rafts paddling into the surf in Borneo. Packing a bunch of big sailboats in a tiny stream was a good way to make that exciting carnage happen again. At the five-minute announcement prior to the start, Nellie and I had decided together that we would prefer to finish marking our maps (plotting coordinates and sketching route lines) and start a little late instead of starting on time and then having to pause later for more marking. Plus, we reckoned, that'd keep us out of the initial chaos when the gun went off.

Patience is paying off, I thought to myself as boats crashed and people yelled while we calmly marked the maps and organized gear before slowly pushing off about five minutes late, And we should probably keep that in mind throughout the race. Take care of ourselves now so we can keep moving consistently later on.

Estimates from the map had us sailing the camakau about forty-three miles on this first stretch. We'd paddle down a gradually growing river for about ten miles to the ocean—hopefully long enough to get the paddling and steering dialed in—before hitting the open ocean, where locals had assured us the wind was always blowing and we'd be able to hoist the sail and cruise right along, propelled by the wind. We may have started last, but paddling the big, slow boat down that river we soon found ourselves in the middle of the pack. Shane's expert steering from the stern (back) of the craft kept us going straight while other teams zigged and zagged. Nellie sat in front of Shane, then Dad near the mast and me at the bow (front). The biggest challenge early on, in fact, was the wake generated by a motorboat full of cameras that accelerated spasmodically as it tried to stay just in front of us. Any doubts that most of our trip would be filmed evaporated (unlike our sweat, which quickly became a slimy coating in the thick humidity), and we eased into life in front of the camera, reality-TV style. I had been filmed in many races over the years, but when a camera only goes to you occasionally, it's natural to try and come up with something funny or inspiring or interesting to say. When *everything* is filmed and recorded, for more than a week, I was learning, you might as well just be yourself and forget about the cameras. As conversations inevitably led to the full-on potty talk and sailor-mouths common to any long excursion in the wilderness, we'd sometimes find ourselves laughing about the Amazon interns who'd have to listen to all of our audio months later in some sound room in LA or New York; they'd think we were nuts, for sure!

A few hours of hard work had us, finally, out into the ocean. The top teams were already out of sight, but a slew of others were way behind us. We were working together well. Every so often, in unison with our paddle strokes, Shane would chant, "Hup, hup, HO!" That last one was the signal to shift from paddling on one side of the boat to the other. This was pretty simple—for those who didn't have Alzheimer's. We were all smiles, though, and more than once the team got a chuckle out of missed exchanges or Dad's comments like, "Shane, what the hell are you talking about?! What's the deal with all this chanting?! The Stray Dogs used to just paddle on one side the whole time…no whining allowed or energy wasted changing sides!"

At the first of dozens of official checkpoints along the course, we washed onto a tropical island beach, where I jumped out and brought our passport to the race official, who initialed the appropriate lines. The race was barely underway, but in this case we'd already spent hours under the hot sun, so Shane ran over to a tiny shop and bought a round of Cokes. We soon found a camera in our faces, and I tried to briefly share our strategy of keeping it steady, working patiently (as fast as we can, as slow as we must), and, likely, sleeping quite a bit—even on the first night. It seemed like some of the race staff were surprised to see us making it this far—let alone doing so ahead of half the field—but everyone was positive and incredibly supportive, particularly the locals.

At this point in the long day of paddling, the wind had yet to blow, and we had pretty much resigned ourselves to paddling many more hours en route to another island, where we'd trek 13 miles up and over a mountain, likely in the dark.

First, though, came navigating the reefs.

If you've ever looked closely at a detailed ocean map (that's what we Coloradoans usually call a nautical chart), you'll see a lot more than blue for water. There are symbols, tide notes, depth indicators, markers for buoys and reefs, and a whole bunch of other stuff I was trying to learn yet again, on the fly, while paddling the same watercraft used by ancients to colonize the Pacific. Nellie and I had done pretty well so far in taking and keeping compass bearings; thankfully, the islands on the map were matching up with the ones we paddled past. When it came to avoiding reefs, however, we gradually realized there'd probably be some guessing and last-minute dodging.

The Fijians take their coral reefs seriously—and for

good reason. Bleaching constantly degrades reefs around the world, and Fiji has not escaped. The country bans sunscreen containing chemicals harmful to reefs, and that turns out to be most sunscreens. Plus the race organizers told us sternly that we were *not* to hit any reefs with our camakaus. Hitting a reef, they said, could smash hundreds of years of marine growth—and would likely puncture and sink the boat as well. The message was clear: hit a reef, and your race is probably over. During high tide, the water line was well above the reefs, and looking down on them provided a spectacular view of rainbow color and vibrant sea life.

But now it was low tide, which meant that many reefs were covered by only a few feet of water. And, looking more closely at the nautical chart (I had now started calling it that in my head to build my own confidence), I saw that reefs not only ringed the islands but were also all over the place— even way out here in the ocean! I knew roughly where we were, but I could never really tell if we were right above a marked reef or not. So, I resorted to the only good option for a high-altitude boy out in the Fijian ocean: stand up in the stern to get a slightly better view and yell to Shane if it looked like we were going to hit something! Dad gave me shit for not paddling for about an hour, but he passed on my offer to let him stand up and rely on his balance (or lack thereof) to not fall out of the boat.

With me on reef watch, Nellie keeping the bearing, Dad cracking jokes, and Shane steering, paddling, and basically keeping the whole thing moving forward, we finally made it to the next checkpoint at a large island. We anchored our camakau next to the others, knowing we'd return to it after the trek, and trudged through muddy water to the transition area, a little tired from paddling a slow, heavy boat for ten hours but enthused nonetheless and eager to be on our feet.

We'd made it through one segment of the race, and it was clear to all that Mace meant business!

Well, he meant business until checkpoint staff started chatting him up, and then storytelling-cussing-joking mode was back. Dad shooting the shit with whoever was around—and if he was around, so were they, flocking to the smiling old guy—was actually a pretty good fit at the transition areas because it left the rest of us to focus on refilling bottles, marking new maps, changing gear in and out, making meals, and strategizing. Shane is the fastest transitioner I have ever seen (huge compliment in the weird little world of adventure racing), but I noticed he was just a little slow at this first shift from paddling to trekking.

"Geez, Shane, did you drop a hot skillet on your lap or something?"

"I'm a little sunburned here, Trav...little sunburned."

I'd known the bright red all over his upper and inner quads was sunburn, and my comment was mostly a buddy-to-buddy rub about the tight, short "Euro shorts" Shane liked to sport. Those had been team-issued years ago when Shane raced on Team Buff, a top crew on the international circuit captained by the one and only Emma Roca.

Known around the world as an adventure racing world champion and ultrarunner with podium finishes at UTMB, Hardrock, Leadville, Run Rabbit Run (all prestigious and highly competitive), Emma and her family had become close friends with Shane, Nellie, me, and our families. We shed tears together when I told her about Dad's diagnosis via video call, and her loving embrace before the race made it clear that we were in this thing together. Her Team Summit would likely be days ahead of us out on the course, but Andrew might be able to collaborate with David, Emma's husband and TAC, and we'd both be asking for updates about our friends at the checkpoints.

It looked like Shane's sunburn would probably blister, but he pulled up those Euros a little bit to prevent rubbing (and later ended up going commando in some baggier pants for most of the race) and hit the trail running. Bottles filled and bags packed, we headed up the trail after Shane, ready for about thirteen miles on foot that would take us a couple thousand feet up and over a jungly mountain.

Hiking down the road as darkness hit for the first time this race, we noticed that four racers had become five. A cameraman was present.

Athletic. Fit. Experienced. Dude is ready to roll.

Athletes can't help but assess those around them on the course, and my initial impressions of this guy behind the lens were positive. He was cruising right along with us, silently focusing the small, expensive HD video camera on Dad. As the miles passed and Camera Guy kept rollin'—both the film and his legs—I started to think this was probably a full-on embedded reporter gig, Anderson Cooper–style.

"What's your name and where are you from?"

"Jochen. Germany." His English was good enough; the smile, nothing but sincere.

"Jochen, welcome to Team Endure!"

Embedded camerapeople had joined us in previous races. They aren't allowed to help in any way, but when you trek for days through challenging conditions with someone, I figure it's only proper to help them feel welcome—and to help them perform as a positive force that doesn't drag the team down. That in mind, I really did mean that Jochen was now part of the team. As it turned out, he'd be with us for all of the trekking on this course. Between foot sections, he'd connect with a local driver and move ahead to the next trek, often taking detours to say hi to us on the way while we paddled or biked, encouraging us with his smile and gathering more valuable footage. Yup, Jochen was now on the team, and we all appreciate the true friendship that developed over hours of conversation and shared struggle that week.

There'd be time for fun for sure, but on that first night, Jochen had one primary challenge: keep up with Dad as he absolutely hammered up the steep, muddy, rooty trail climbing from the coast to the peak. In fact, Shane, Nellie, and I were also pushing pretty hard to hang with the pace Dad was setting! Most mountain athletes like us try to survive the ocean stuff so we can battle back on foot and bike; Dad was clearly at home climbing this mountain. Conditioned through decades of high-altitude running, snowshoeing, and mountain biking, Dad's sixty-five-year-old heart, lungs, and legs were in prime condition. Maybe he couldn't tie his shoes or read the map or drive a car, but Dad was smashing this thing. Peering through the salty sweat in my eyes, I let my headlamp rest on Dad's powerful calves, flexing and releasing as they lifted him through the dark jungle. The exertion was challenging and the uncertainty was high, but my smile was big, just as it was thirty years ago hammering up that washboard dirt road in Evergreen looking at those same calves.

Having passed a number of teams on the climb, including some who'd gone out too fast and were now paying a price with vomiting and dehydration, we checked in at the summit, inquiring briefly about our friends ahead. Emma, Mike, Josiah, Nathan—they were all looking good at the front of the pack, so at 10:00 p.m. on a starlit night from a windy Fijian outlook... life was as it should be.

We continued along the ridgeline and headed downhill, back toward the boats. And immediately slowed down. Way down.

Descending, it turned out, was much harder than climbing due to the visual-spatial challenges of Alzheimer's.

Dad's balance had declined, and even during the day-light, challenges with depth perception made hills look much steeper than they actually were. Dad and I had discussed this during training; terrain that he had run and biked over for years now appeared deadly. Things were even worse in the dark, where Dad's vision strug-gled to track the headlamp's beam and make sense of the dynamic interplay of many lights on rocks, roots, mud, puddles, branches, and leaves. I knew a fall on this down-hill jungle hike was unlikely to injure anyone badly, but I also knew Dad's perception was that it was incredibly dangerous, maybe even deadly (which it was not). In a true example of his courage, belief in himself, and trust in his teammates, Dad continued forward, moving as quickly as he could while grabbing trees, sliding frequently, and falling often. We all knew about these limitations, and no one was upset when a couple teams cruised past. We became a unit: pointing out hand and foot placements amongst the mud and rocks, bracing each other on drops, taking Dad's trek-king poles when he needed to grab trees and then handing them back when they could be used. This experience was teaching me a new depth of teamwork. Writing this almost two years later, I am deeply thankful for that new under-standing and rite of passage as Dad and I traded roles in our relationship. I continually rely on this insight and growth as we continue to wade together through the unknown of Alzheimer's.

Having finished the trek and in doing so confirmed to ourselves and those around us that we were here to get this thing done, we arrived back at the transition area where we'd left the boats at about midnight. As teams around us rushed back to the boats to hammer through the night, we found a quiet spot on the grass, laid out our tarp, cooked an evening meal (dehydrated something or other…yum!), and lay down to sleep. Our goal was to be back in the camakau just after the 6:00 a.m. sunrise.

Like everyone, I've got many ongoing challenges: anxiety, depression, perfectionism, thinking my mustache is cool. The list goes on. Thankfully, trouble sleeping is not on it. If you're going to lie down, I figure, you might as well sleep. And that's just what I did, all night long on that tarp on the grass on a Fijian island.

Dad and I had sandwiched ourselves between Shane and Nellie. The thinking was that if Dad woke up disoriented someone would hear him and be able to help.

Shane broke the news as I fired up the stove for coffee and dehydrated eggs: "I woke up last night and Mace was gone."

I lost focus and almost set my map on fire. "No shit! What do you mean, dude?!"

"Well, I was standing there peeing and realized we were a man down. I shined my headlamp around and found him over there by the porta-potties." Calm, patient, and helpful as always, Shane brought Dad back to our sleeping area, helped him lie down, and stayed awake until he heard him snoring again.

Dad didn't remember anything in the morning, but I took this seriously, noting darkness as our primary foe for three reasons:

> 1. It was clear that our pace would be much slower in the dark.
> 2. If Dad was awake and it was dark out, there was a good chance disorientation might come knocking.
> 3. With twelve hours of darkness in every

twenty-four at this equatorial latitude, we'd
have to hustle during the day and make very
few mistakes to stay ahead of the time cutoffs.

And now, about twenty-four hours into the race, the
first cutoff was only thirty hours away and on the other side
of more camakau, a long stand-up paddle (SUP), and a very
challenging mountain bike ride. I knew from experience that
looking at the enormity of the course ahead could potentially
be overwhelming, but given the circumstances it was imperative to forecast well in advance, largely in the interest of hitting a good place to sleep—like a village or aid station and not
out in the rainy jungle—shortly after sundown.

Other than the brief and potentially dangerous cap-
size incident I related in the introduction to this book, the
camakau journey back to mainland went pretty well. At the
midafternoon transition from sailing to stand-up paddling,
we passed a few teams who had raced all night. The six-hour
"delay" to sleep was already made up, simply because we
could move in a straighter line on the water with daylight.
After thirty-six hours without sleep in the heat and humidity, some of these teams were pretty wasted: some slept on
the grass and others wandered aimlessly. Dad, however, was
fresh and stoked for more. His back and shoulders hurt, but
that was nothing new.

Sleeping also helped Nellie and me to nail the navigation, and we successfully SUPed from the beach, across a
big bay, and to the correct small creek among a few choices.
Finding the right creek sounds easy enough, but one of the
top US teams, which happened to contain our good friends
Mike Kloser, Josiah Middaugh, and Gretchen Reeves, had
previously turned into the wrong creek and lost more than
five hours. From there we'd SUP about eighteen miles up the

creek to a small village where our bikes were waiting in boxes to be assembled and ridden.

Team Endure continued to lean heavily on Shane, who set the pace, provided recommendations on our form, and even towed his teammates along with a thin bungee line from one SUP to another. A few hours into this journey, heat changed rapidly to cold when a storm blew in. In adventure races, you're usually too hot or too cold, and even Fiji was no exception.

Approaching a bridge, we made a decision that led to one of the strangest and most fun things I have ever done. Freezing in the rain and with Dad's back beginning to seize from paddling, we opted to take out at the bridge and trek along a road to the next transition area. We'd be walking about five miles instead of SUPing eight. This sounds like an easy trade—except that we'd have to carry the heavy SUPs along with us!

Shane and I had previously been bold about carrying the SUPs.

"Think we can carry those things, Trav?"

"Yeah, we'll just deflate three of them and stack them on top of the inflated one. Then you and I will put them on top of our heads and walk. Simple."

"Are you guys sure about that? They seem pretty heavy to me." Nellie was skeptical. Right, as well. I had to walk less than ten strides with those things on my head to realize that five miles of it was sure to rupture every disc in my neck and back. The weight was simply too much.

We shrugged off the SUPs and went back to the drawing board. By this time, our circus—dragging SUPs out of the water, shivering in the rain, changing clothes, yelling to each other in the downpour—had drawn quite a crowd of locals. We had the best gear made and were struggling in the weather; they seemed to be comfortable and easygoing in jorts, T-shirts, and bare feet, behaving as if it were another sunny day.

Dragging the SUPs five miles would surely shred them, and we were just about to begin reinflating them for the upstream paddle when a local guy rushed in. "Guys, I have a wheelbarrow. Would you like to borrow it?"

"Heck yeah, buddy!" Shane hugged the guy and ran to his house with him.

Before we knew it, we were trekking along the hilly, dirt road with a wheelbarrow from (I estimated) about 1947. Old and rusty, but super solid. Shane pushed the wheelbarrow full of four deflated SUPs. I pulled it with a bungee cord attached to my waist. Dad carried the paddles and Nellie walked next to him with the PFDs (life jackets). And our temporary teammates, a couple of teenage boys, walked with us, having come along to bring the wheelbarrow back when we were done with it. They seemed to think nothing of this ten-mile hike in bare feet over a rocky road in the rain that would surely end well into the night. The boys were athletic, energetic, and enthusiastic. They threw rocks at the enormous, raven-sized bats that flew by ("We can eat those") and carried machetes ("In case the wild pig attacks").

Those five miles of hilly trekking while pulling a wheelbarrow with my friends and my dad made for a few of my best hours of racing. Ever. I wasn't hammering for a win, but I was present and happy. Shane's muscles bulged as he carried that thing over the bumps. Dad and Nellie became one, stepping stride for stride as she asked him question after question about the good old days of adventure racing and his legal career and his family. She had realized that disorientation started creeping in as soon as darkness hovered—and also that Dad's focus could stay with us if he was engaged in conversation. From then on, the two old friends were a pair every evening until we found a place to sleep. It was the epitome of teamwork, and it was beautiful. The boys ran along, walking and chatting with us for a while before sprinting back into the jungle in chase of a bat or to cut down another coconut to share with us.

An hour later at the transition area from SUPing to biking, heaven had become hell.

"Travis, you gotta tell me what the fuck is going on here!"

"We're at the transition area in a village in Fiji, Dad. Let's go sleep in that school over there and start biking again in the morning."

"What the hell, Trav?! Did you even pay the entry fee for this damn race? And why the fuck are you and Nellie charging these teams to sleep in this hotel?"

Dad's been mad at me about five times in my life. Now he was pissed. I hadn't seen this rage since the '94 Mosquito Massacre in Alaska. (That's kind of funny now; gotta have a little humor, even—and especially—when things are serious, but at the moment I was scared as shit.)

I knew Dad was disoriented and I had the presence of mind not to take his words personally. Nonetheless, I ripped off my Amazon microphone because I had no idea where this was going. The darkness, bright headlamps everywhere, noises of a village, and many languages back and forth were clearly too much for Alzheimer's at this moment.

"We gotta sleep," I whispered to Shane and Nellie. "If we can't sleep or if things aren't better in the morning, I'm pulling the plug on this thing."

The brain is a funny thing. I can feel totally overwhelmed by parenting or work or even just organizing my garage. But now, in the middle of the night out in the jungle during what could be shaping up to be a real medical emergency, one part of my mind raced while another stayed calm and focused.

Get Dad to sleep and reevaluate in the morning.

The focus was clear, and amidst his questioning and confusion ("Why'd you try to steal that guy's bike back there, Trav?!"), I focused on the goal and got us into the school and to a calm spot in the corner of a classroom. The concrete floor was hard, but I made Dad as comfortable as possible with a PFD under his head and a space blanket over his body. Uncertain speech gradually became snoring.

Lying next to Dad with tears in my eyes and my head on my own PFD and my hand on top of his (out of love, and to make sure he didn't leave while I slept), I finally fell asleep with absolutely no idea what would happen in the morning.

A mile at a time, Trav... a mile at a time.

Cut from the baseball team in seventh grade.

"Keep the faith, Bud. I believe in you, and I know things will work out."

Can't decide if I should leave the CU-Boulder cross-country and track teams to join the triathlon team. Stressed about the choice.

"Keep the faith, Bud. I believe in you, and I know things will work out."

Only halfway through the 24 Hours of Moab mountain bike race and already totally shattered.

"Keep the faith, Bud. I believe in you, and I know things will work out."

Struggling with the uncertainty of quitting my teaching job and principal licensure program to become a self-employed athlete and coach.

"Keep the faith, Bud. I believe in you, and I know things will work out."

Night two of a ten-night race and things are already looking really bad here in Fiji. What the hell was I thinking, anyway?!

"Keep the faith, Bud. I believe in you, and I know things will work out." (He didn't say it this time, but I remembered and told myself.)

"Good morning, Dad. How are you?" His answer would likely determine our fate, I figured. I didn't want to go home but knew we might have to.

"Man, Bud, I feel pretty good." He rubbed his face and then smiled, blue eyes beaming again. "Sorry about last night...I really thought you and Danelle were running some sort of underground business. That was weird!"

"Yeah, no shit it was weird, Dad."

"And we are actually signed up for the race, right?"

"We sure are. I'm glad things are better than last night. I was scared."

"Me too, Bud. Thanks for helping me. I love you."

"I love you too, Dad."

Sleep is incredible, and it was clear that Dad was a new guy. And it was also fascinating that he remembered the disorientation of the night before. We talked through the previous day and the weird night. Dad knew we were in the race and what we were doing—and that he was stoked for coffee and food. The local women had washed our jerseys overnight and now served all-you-can-eat homemade *babakau* (imagine the tastiest fried combination of a pancake and a donut you've ever had). We chowed down, hopped on our bikes (Shane and Nellie had built them up in the dark while Dad and I slept before hitting the hay themselves), and rolled out of town to enthusiastic chants of "Bula, bula, bula!" from men, women, and children. The race was back on for Team Endure!

And it sure as hell was time to race because we'd have to cover about twenty-five miles on the bike over steep, hilly terrain in order to make the first cutoff at 1:00 p.m. that afternoon. Team Stray Dogs rolled out with us, and it was great to share some miles with them before Dad lowered the hammer on a long, steep climb. His fitness and pace were amazing! We quickly dropped the other riders, which was fine because I knew Shane and Nellie could descend much faster as soon as the road turned downhill again. The old guy who was totally disoriented last night and needed help putting on his jersey this morning was now riding uphill faster than all but the most elite in the race. If adventure racing with Dad has taught me one thing, it's that even when things look really bad, they don't always necessarily get worse. We were having fun again, cranking the climbs and enjoying incredible scenery of limestone cliffs, deep canyons, and virgin jungle as we made our way to Fiji's interior.

Passing team after team, we again fell into a rhythm together as a unit. It's crucial to eat constantly in these races, but Alzheimer's can distort a person's sense of time. Shane took full responsibility for Dad's eating. He'd pedal up next to Dad: "Split a bar with me, Mace?"

"Geez, you guys are force-feeding me! I swear I'm gaining weight!" We'd crack up at what became a team joke.

Shane's Bear Grylls interpretation also popped up

frequently. He'd pop out of the bushes after a pee with an exuberant expression and British accent, mimicking what Bear had said before the race: "Mace, you must finish the race!" We'd roll with laughter...and pedal even more furiously.

Our pace was steady all day. Moving as fast as we could and as slow as we must, we smashed the climbs and crawled down the descents (Alzheimer's significantly impacted Dad's perception of speed, and what would have felt casual to him a few years ago now seemed dangerously fast). Particularly with the looming cutoff, waiting on the descents could have been frustrating for Nellie and Shane, but we were all so committed to the team game that any pauses they may have been forced to make just made for more fun, joking, eating, or prepping another snack for Dad.

Before we knew it, we were pedaling into an enthusiastic crowd backdropped by a few helicopters and a sprawling camp of tents and vehicles. This was Camp 1, and we'd made the first official time cut! A number of teams were not going to make this cutoff, and some of the organizers and crew were clearly surprised to see us.

NINE

*My father-in-law, Mark Pence, is ninety-three
years old and is one of the best people I've
ever known, and I believe he feels similarly
about me. If he outlives me, I can't imagine
how sad this happy man would be.*

*So far I have not told him about my ALZ
simply because of the enormous sadness it would
cause him. I truly hope he never has to know. If he
is around to watch the Eco-Challenge broadcast,
then I will have to tell him before that. I love
him just like my own Dad, and I don't know how
I will tell him that I might die before him.*

—MACE'S JOURNAL

YET ANOTHER REASON adventure racing is good training
for Alzheimer's and other scary things: the sport—like a
serious diagnosis or chronic illness—forces you to continually
do your best amidst the uncertainty of not knowing what's
ahead. Those maps Nellie and I had marked during the
camakau rodeo only got us here, to Camp 1. This was
approximately the first 20 percent of the race, and we
knew nothing about the rest of the course. Now, having
made the first cutoff, we received maps covering Camp 1
to Camp 2, a journey that included trekking, building and
paddling *bilibilis,* and mountain biking. Don't know what
a bilibili is? Neither did I! But I had learned we'd have
about 35 hours (from the afternoon of day three to late in

the night on day four) to do all of that before the next cut-off at Camp 3.

This transition area at Camp 1 provided the first place for teams to see their Team Assistance Crew (TAC). We were pumped to see Andrew's smiling face—and he was downright ecstatic to see ours! In two and a half days of racing, Dad, Shane, Nellie, and I had established a rhythm and accumulated some fatigue. But Andrew was fresh, and this made for his first moment of actually "racing" with us, so his enthusiasm provided a welcome boost to the team. By the time we'd washed away a couple days of grime in the crystal-line river running through camp, Andrew had cleaned our bikes, tuned them up, and completed about half of the map marking. Wow, talk about service!

About an hour later, with the Camp 1 cutoff looming, we got another good surprise: Team Stray Dogs! Dr. Bob was quite ill in the stomach, likely from some jungle-borne virus or bacteria, and even his decades of work as a renowned pathologist didn't seem to be helping with diagnosis or treatment. All over sixty, the Stray Dogs had persevered as a unit to make a challenging cutoff that many athletes half their age had missed. We had come into the race with a mind-set that, although they might not actually be together on the course, Team Endure and Team Stray Dogs were really one extended group. We were pumped that they'd made the first cutoff, and the older contingent really was showing that aging athletes can continue to perform as the decades pass.

After on-camera interviews with the Amazon Prime Video production crew and a hot, tasty meal prepared by Andrew, we were ready to head out, this time on foot en route to another small village where we'd get on the river.

Typically, Coloradoans like us think of fun river-rafting trips when we think "get on the river." Where I live, in

Salida, Colorado, most families own at least one river craft or another, and the summer culture centers around rafting day trips and overnight trips. In summers past, my family and I have rafted in Colorado and Utah with Shane and his family and Nellie and hers. One time we even joined Emma Roca and her family for a wonderful float down the Animas River near Durango, Colorado, where Shane lives. The rapids were fun; the smiles were big; the boats buoyant, stable, and safe.

Here in Fiji, after trekking all afternoon and into the evening, we now found ourselves getting ready for a river trip on boats that clearly were not buoyant, stable, safe—or even constructed! In fact, the "boats" were just huge piles of bamboo poles when we got to them. The Fjiian bilibili is a traditional raft composed of bamboo poles tied together with rope or twine. It's about ten feet long and four feet wide. Imagine Huck Finn pushing his way down the Mississippi on a sketchy, homemade rig, propelled along with a long pole in the style of a gondolier in Venice. Well, that would be us soon—but on a Fijian river full of rocks and wave trains, in the dark. But first we had to build the things.

When the Prime Video coverage aired months later, we discovered that our friend Emma, then over a full day ahead of us, had captured that bilibili-building scene the best. In episode 2 of "World's Toughest Race: Eco-Challenge Fiji" we see Emma going strong in fifth place—just as vibrant and energetic as the Fijian children around her—working hand in hand with the locals to construct two bilibilis that Team Summit would paddle and pole for the next twelve hours. "My goodness," Emma says to the Fijian kids helping her, "You are strong! *Muy bien!*" Her contagious enthusiasm and sincere spirit shine through as she turns to the camera: "I love to suffer and do this sport and finish the race. But, above all, you need these experiences with these locals because you are on a fantastic island with wonderful people who perhaps you might not see again." Emma captures the spirit of Eco-Challenge here: humans moving across the landscape as they evolved to do, working as a team, in harmony with friends and teammates and locals. She was full of life and harnessing the moment.

Later on at the same village, Shane and Nellie coordinated a late-night bilibili build while Dad, Jochen, and I made some dinner. As I said, Jochen was officially the camera guy, but he had become part of the crew and was very thoughtful and intuitive about engaging Dad in conversation that kept him tuned in and oriented. This of course made for footage that could be used later in production, but it was also sincerely friendly and helpful to our mission.

At about midnight, with the bilibilis constructed and waiting for us by the river, we walked into the village seeking shut-eye. Teams around us would surely push through without stopping, but we knew that real sleep—in a warm, dry building instead of the mud on a riverbank—would have us going steady the next day.

"Hey, friend," Shane said to a young man who had been watching our approach from the edge of the village, "is there somewhere we can sleep here?"

"Bula! Yes! You come with me to the house of my brother-cousin." Every guy in rural Fiji seems to be everyone else's "brother-cousin."

Where in America or Europe (or anywhere) can you walk into town in the middle of the night and be welcomed into a stranger's house? Well, you sure can in Fiji.

Nice and simple and loving. That's how the house was. A woman gave us pancakes and hot tea, and we sat with her and the kids, exchanging smiles. One open room, a bamboo floor mat, not much else. Bathroom out back. Sensing a universal spirit of love that must be shared by all humans over time and can almost be touched if you look in the right places (the same thing Emma speaks of in the TV program), I fell asleep, smiling, next to my dad, three good friends, and a pile of little kids.

Our goal was to hit the river at 5:30 a.m., and the alarm went off an hour before that. Third morning of this, and the routine was set: fire up stove (hopefully without burning myself; liquid fuel is dicey), hot coffee, dehydrated meal, help Dad dress, "Split a bar, Mace?," hit the road.

Early morning on the river was cold and dark. Adventure races often include "dark zones," or segments of the course that are closed when it's dark outside. These typically occur on whitewater segments like the river rafting we'd be doing later in this race. The bilibili section we were now starting did not have a dark zone because most of the river was nice and calm, but shortly after putting in at the village, we encountered some small wave trains and dangerous strainers (dams of logs, sticks, and other refuse that can flip and puncture boats or trap a person's foot). Even in the dark, this water would have been easy with a raft or kayak. But these bamboo rafts, we were discovering, weren't modern rafts or kayaks! Not even close.

They sank halfway into the river, submerging your butt if you were sitting (as Dad was most of the time) or your feet if you were standing (like the rest of us). A practiced paddler can turn a river kayak on a dime or dig in to accelerate it quickly around an obstacle; these bilibilis required a good long distance to turn and seemed to have just one speed: slow.

Paddling along in the bilibili with Dad in the front and me behind, my mind wandered back to my first time in a two-person inflatable kayak with him. I was probably about twelve, and as we navigated rapids in the Arkansas River near Buena Vista, Colorado, I hooted and hollered, oblivious to the dangers from which Dad's skilled paddling sheltered me. Now, with our roles reversed, I sensed and then saw a strainer coming quickly at us out of the dark, river right. I dug hard to turn our "boat," but I could immediately tell we were turning too slowly.

Shit! If we hit that strainer the race could be over... or worse. I didn't say it, but I thought it and imagined the bilibili exploding into shreds and both of us floundering in the wave train.

"Paddle hard, Dad!" I did say that, and he did it. I knew it hurt his back, but screw that. This was do or die, here and now.

We missed the strainer by about an inch and floated on, into the darkness.

"Man, Bud, that was fun! Nice work."

"Fun? Shit, Dad, that was a close call. Yeah... I guess it was kind of fun though. Way to paddle, Dad."

"Way to steer, Bud."

A partner trade had Dad and Shane paddling together with the former managing increasingly significant back and shoulder issues while the latter powered and steered from the stern. Nellie and I took the other bilibili, which had a serious proclivity for tracking to the right, and we tried to keep up for the next thirteen hours while constantly using steering strokes to turn left. Have you ever thought about paddling a bilibili for fourteen hours in a muddy river through the jungle? Well, don't, because it's not very fun.

Now well into the afternoon on day 4, we finally dragged the heavy bamboo rafts out of the river and up a steep incline at the takeout. This segment of the race had been taxing, and we were all feeling the paddling after doing mostly that for three out of four days. The second cutoff loomed at Camp

2, and we now rebuilt our bikes and hopped on for another thirty miles of very hilly mountain biking to get there.

Dad was back in his element, hammering the hills yet again, but I could tell his back was getting worse. Shane and I took some weight on our bikes and packs to relieve Dad's back, and each time we stopped I rubbed Biofreeze gel on his back and shoulders. It helped a bit. We knew ibuprofen would feel even better, but that was out of the question since he had only one kidney.

Hours passed and darkness fell. We had top-of-the-line bike light systems, but dark is dark, especially when Alzheimer's is present. The pace slowed dramatically, and minor disorientation had Dad talking about a big concert up ahead put on by race director Kevin Hodder and a bunch of bands. Oh, man, we gotta get there and go to sleep soon, I thought to myself. In the dark, on poorly marked roads through a big river valley, I knew we were going the right way but struggled to tell how far we had to go. Nothing to do now but pedal onward into the unknown, a mile at a time.

Sometime around midnight, the camp finally materialized ahead, and we rode in through torches and clapping to a warm crowd and high fives from Andrew, Heather Ulrich, Jochen, race staff, and locals. We'd made cutoff two of five and completed roughly 40 percent of the World's Toughest Race. If anyone had doubted Mace at the start, they were now convinced: the old guy with Alzheimer's is still the real deal. We headed to our tents for some shut-eye.

"Man, Andrew, is this the rockiest campsite in the whole place?"

"Nope, Mace, I actually gave you the flattest spot around."

We all chuckled. This field seemed to be populated by rock-hard basketballs under a thin layer of dirt and grass.

Nonetheless, sleep is sleep, and we were glad to be in our own tents and sleeping bags, which Andrew had prepared in advance. Dad woke once during the night to visit one of the porta-potties on the edge of the camp and then couldn't find our tents amongst so many others, but a local guy supporting the event noticed him and helped him find his way. Adventure racing is a team sport, and so is life.

After another solid sleep, we rolled out of Camp 2 on our bikes. The sun had just risen on day 5. At the beginning of an expedition, the body and mind are not quite comfortable with primal, outdoor life, but by now we were fully engaged in a feral mode of existence: keep eating, keep drinking, help each other, move, navigate the land with which you are now one, to hell with cleanliness—splashing in rivers is enough. It felt good, comfortable, real...alive. I truly believe humans evolved to move through the landscape like this; events like Eco-Challenge really just give us a chance to reconnect with what we're meant to be. Did the wise elder of a hunter-gatherer band get left behind just because he was slowing down or not quite as sharp? I doubt it, and I was becoming more and more comfortable embracing my new role as the next leader. Doing hard things is good, and it's important to practice the navigation of uncertainty. As Dad always says, "It's all good mental training." I could tell that bashing around in this jungle was doing me some good, and my mindset felt far away from drinking too much and smashing shovels on trees, thank goodness.

And, philosophical thinking aside, the race was back on, big-time. A number of teams like ours at the rear of the pack were now close together, and we knew we'd have to race hard—and help each other, teammates or not—to make the next cutoff in two days' time. Before that: another 40 miles of biking in the mud, a short trek, river rafting, and a long trek through the heart of the rugged mountains. Stray Dogs had once again made the cutoff, Marsh, Dr. Bob, Adrian, and Nancy continuing to persevere after many younger teams had dropped out. Pumped to be out there with our friends, we pedaled through long river valleys bordered by high limestone cliffs and virgin jungle.

I've never been one for religion, and concepts like "ask and you shall receive" have always seemed a little naive to me. On the other hand, a couple of weeks with the Fijian people had me sensing an almost palpable interconnectedness, a sense of love that crosses languages and oceans and times, and might even be expressed in basically the same way through the current "religions" and past "mythologies" (and isn't the difference between the two in the eye of the beholder?). Pondering such thoughts and more, I realized we had now been out of drinking water for long enough to generate some concern. For most of this race, we'd been splashing in and out of lowland creeks every few minutes, and it was easy to fill our filter-flasks and sip away. But now we were pedaling a few thousand feet above sea level and hadn't seen a creek for a long time. Just as I thought, Boy, it sure would be nice to get a drink, there it was: a water bottle lying in the mud in front of me! I picked it up. Full. Sniffed. No odor. Sipped. Tasty. Passed it around.

The water bottle in the trail probably fell off another team's bike, but, who knows, maybe it did come from above. Or maybe Jeff Bezos had a satellite cam on us and drones that could swing in to make things happen, *Hunger Games*–style. We had been joking for days about him secretly listening to us (likely from a spaceship) via the microphone around my neck. Either way, that bottle was a nice pickup for all of us. I got a giggle a couple hours later when I surged ahead and out of sight to unpack my secret present for the team: a big bag of

Doritos and a single can of Fanta. I'd bought them hours ago in a village and carried them unseen until just the right time.

"Hey, Dad, look what I just found out here in the jungle!" I held them up as he pushed his bike toward me through the mud. Did I mention the thick, claylike mud that was now above our ankles? And after we had been pushing and carrying the bikes uphill for a few hours since riding them was completely impassable?

"No way! How'd that stuff get out here in the jungle, Bud?"

"Just kidding. I carried it."

Looking back, this wasn't really that funny, but at the time all four of us were a little loopy—probably from low blood sugar and hours of pushing bikes through the mud—and we all cracked up while shoving chips in our faces and luxuriating in a whole three ounces (approximately) of warm soda apiece.

As viewers of *World's Toughest Race: Eco-Challenge Fiji* on Amazon Prime would see, that "biking" section through the mud was pretty epic. The distance was nothing incredible, but the steep, relentless climb and thick, sticky mud were truly daunting. I was able to ride a few short, intermittent downhills here and there, sliding from side to side like I was riding a wild donkey down a toboggan run. Dad tried to ride a few times and quickly crashed. Heck, he was crashing all over the place just pushing his bike. Thankfully the speed was slow and the squishy landings were forgiving. Nonetheless, they pounded his shoulders and back, and I could tell the constant pain was intensifying.

We tried to help each other as much as possible, but the mud-covered bikes each weighed well over fifty pounds and the best we could do for Dad was to frequently dig our muddy fingers between the frame and the wheels so they could actually spin again. Dad's called that stuff "Moab mud" forever, and it's extremely successful at getting absolutely everywhere and ruining the top-of-the-line components we cycling enthusiasts take pride in. My bike had stopped shifting gears hours ago, and only the front brakes were functioning. The progress was slow and challenging, and Dad's on-camera comment, later used by Amazon in promoting the TV program, pretty much summed it up: "*This* is the Eco-Challenge way: either do it or go home."

Finally, late in the afternoon, we looked ahead to see a man with a camera sliding down the hill toward us. Jochen! And if Jochen was walking down the trail, it meant the road at the top of the trail must not be too far away. Coming out of that mud felt like finally getting out of the trenches on the Western Front, and Jochen embraced us as if we'd survived a battle. That's a bit of exaggeration, of course, but the day had been quite strenuous and we were glad to find ourselves approaching the next transition area, where we'd disassemble our bikes, pack them in boxes, and start trekking to the start of the rafting section. My bike box included a soggy note: "Andrew, nothing works on my bike. Umm... see if you can fix it?!" I got a giggle out of imagining him opening the box and finding the half-decomposed paper while overwhelmed by the fumes, nasty bike shorts, and all-consuming grunge within.

Trekking for a few intimate and conversational hours with an Italian team brought us to the rim above a deep canyon through which we'd be whitewater rafting. It was now about 10:00 p.m., and we could not begin rafting until daybreak due to the dark zone for safety. The rafting would occur on one of Fiji's few commercial whitewater rivers, and a small rafting company had set up shop here at the canyon rim. While Shane jogged down the hill to get dibs on one of the roofed tent platforms in the jungle so we'd have a flat, dry place to sleep, Dad, Nellie, and I took some time to shoot the shit with a bunch of local guys who were hanging out there. In a rich, humorous, and real conversation, we asked each other's names and more. Some of these guys had been on the course in 2002 when the Eco went through, and they were pumped to see us back. One of them even recognized Nellie, who had been on a leading team that year.

Although I had a beard and long hair (something about preparing for a week in the jungle had encouraged me to ease into Grunge Mode months in advance; "mental training," I told my unimpressed wife), one guy noticed that Dad and I looked a lot alike.

"You are his son?"

We affirmed. They applauded.

"How old are you?" he asked Dad.

"Me...?" Dad hesitated. "Man, that's a good question! How old am I, Trav?!" We all giggled.

"You're sixty-five, Dad."

"Oh, sixty-five! You strong man, Mace. You finish the race!"

They really got a kick out of Dad's age, and soon each of us had shared our ages, those in their twenties, sixties, and seventies receiving "oohs" and "ahs" for impressive youth and wisdom. I happily eased away for a few minutes so Dad could keep joking around and laughing with his peers. Maybe Alzheimer's generates a need for support around the house. Maybe it presents limitations on things like driving, putting on a climbing harness, doing math, fixing a bike, or getting dressed. Maybe it generates stress and anxiety about the future and what's to come. I know it has for our family. But when it's hard to remember the past and anticipate the future, there's still the present. Right here. Right now. Dad's spirit, his enthusiasm, his happiness and sincere interest in chatting with these old Fijian guys who were just as stoked to chat with him were teaching me to be present; that it's never too late to help someone else; that a man can ask for help and put his trust in family and friends (and even strangers, in Fiji) and still be a real man; that good can almost always be found if you look hard enough for it. Needless to say, the intimate evening with the locals by the rafting shack remains one of the highlights of my Fijian experience.

On top of a hard tent platform under a loud metal roof out in the jungle, I slept well that night as a rainstorm pounded above the roaring river below. Dad awoke at one point, thinking he was in a snowstorm in Detroit (being forced to move back to Detroit has long been a recurring nightmare for him). Luckily, Shane woke up as well and was again able to reorient Dad and help him find sleep.

A few hours later, we navigated possibly the most scenic part of the course as our whitewater raft meandered down a narrow, deep, limestone canyon decorated by spraying waterfalls, chirping birds, and lush plant life. Shane steered our raft expertly, and we all enjoyed the float. We knew the upcoming trek would present an intense chase to stay in the race (by beating the coming cutoff the next day), but for now we were having fun and taking it in.

"Mace," Shane broke the silence, "what's the *one thing* we should know about life?" I don't know if Shane had watched *City Slickers* recently, but it was a well-timed line for sure.

Dad didn't hesitate: "Guys, you must spend as much time with your family as you possibly can." We floated on under the Fijian sun, nodding, smiling, thinking of our spouses and kids, until Dad broke the silence: "I hope my grandchildren remember me as the person I actually am."

"They will, Dad. I promise, Dad. I'll make sure of it, Dad."

As we hit the next rapid, whitewater spray mixed with my tears.

Trekking over tricky jungle trails—narrow, muddy, slippery—in the ensuing section, the race was on. For Team Endure, this segment presented the greatest challenge yet. We'd been going for six days and had about twenty-four hours to make the next cutoff at Camp 3. Dad's back problems were worsening fast, and my calculations of our progress over the unknown terrain had us hitting Camp 3 not long before the cutoff if we pressed hard through the night. But we knew trekking all night without sleep was a recipe for disaster, as was lying down to rest in the mud and rain. Basically, we'd have to keep going until we arrived at a remote village that would hopefully offer at least a little warm, dry sleep.

Our team had grown to include a few local "guides" and their small, rugged horses. Race rules indicated that just for this particular trek locals could be paid for their guiding expertise. And it's a good thing, because without the generous, energetic, athletic guys who showed us the way over this particularly confusing mess of crisscrossing trails through the mountains from village to village, we'd probably still be wandering around out there. Our guides were dressed like the wheelbarrow boys: basketball shorts and jerseys, nothing more nor less. As we sheltered under rain jackets and top-of-the-line running shoes with the best sticky rubber made, these guys set a blistering pace in their bare feet, often while carrying one (or more) of our backpacks. They said nothing of the rain, cold, sun, or heat and seemed to need very few calories. Rugged, hardy, and ranging in age from teens to sixties, these guys and their horses were clearly accustomed to spending all day trekking over this challenging terrain.

The condition of the "trail" was now quickly deteriorating. And so was Dad's back. As the hours passed and darkness fell, I fell dozens of times. Dad fell *hundreds* of times. His back was totally jacked, wrenched sideways in pain and spasm. Using poles to support himself, his shoulder was also in agony.

Now the trail kicks up steeply and Dad is sliding backward, into the dark jungle. I reach back, and his hand goes into mine. We go on. The connection, the love, feels the same as it did when I was seven, walking in the dark.

Sloshing through the jungle in the dark, Dad off-balance and basically unable to see the mud, rocks, and bushes, we progressed slowly as a unit. Nellie scouted the path and called obstacles. I followed, supporting Dad from the front while he scrambled along the mud, rocks, and rivers using feet, hands, poles, and sheer determination. Shane rounded out the line, often grabbing Dad's jersey from behind to provide extra support and connecting with Dad and me as we crossed dozens of streams, Dad sandwiched between us with his arms around our shoulders. Having caught up to a couple of other teams, we were now part of a slow-moving, late-night, muddy-jungle caravan composed of athletes, guides, and loud horses that whinnied and neighed as their hooves clanked down the rocky terrain behind us. It was one of those surreal, once-in-a-lifetime marches: nothing to do but move forward through the darkness, minute by minute, step by step, mile by mile.

Dad's balance and vision were off, but the constant change in terrain kept his mind engaged. So did the pain in his back. He was now stopping every few minutes to take on a sort of Downward Dog-ish yoga position that would temporarily lessen the pain and cramping. (Since the race aired, multiple strangers have come up to Dad to tell him they now call that stretch the Mace Pose). The pace was slow and laborious, but there was no chance at all of sleeping in the rain, so we moved on, hoping to finally reach the tiny village marked on the map.

At one point, encouraged by his teammates, Dad agreed to try riding one of the horses, as some of the other athletes had been doing. Particularly with his diminished balance and the technical terrain, we knew there could be some risk here. And within about five seconds of Dad saddling up, the horse spooked, kicking and whinnying.

"Get me down, guys!"

"Shit! No go!"

Shane, the guide, and I braced Dad as he fell off the horse and back to the relative safety of slippery rocks in a river. Back to walking, we were all thankful that the cowboy stunt didn't end a whole lot worse.

Finally, thankfully, we found ourselves in a village at about 1:30 a.m. Given the looming cutoff in less than twelve hours, the teams around us would keep pushing, but we knew we had to sleep. Crawling to bed in another warm and welcoming home surrounded by a generous family and sleepy-eyed kids, Shane summed it up: "Mace, I've seen a lot of crazy shit out there. But you pushing through that was the most impressive thing yet."

Dad didn't hesitate: "I have absolutely no intention of quitting." We all slept soundly, with the only interruption coming when Nellie awoke to discover a small child cuddling next to her for warmth and love. Danelle smiled, gave thanks, thought of her own boys, Noah and Will, and went back to sleep.

Once again under the shining sun, Team Endure was battered but not beaten. After a few more river crossings in the early morning, we finally reached flatter terrain where

Dad could safely mount the horse. An entire village rushed out to help him; Dad enjoyed a back massage from the ladies while the guys created a makeshift saddle and stirrups out of ropes and straps. They were *pumped* for Mace, and he was stoked for them. We strolled out of the village, laughing to ourselves as we sang, "Mamas, don't let your babies grow up to be cowboys!"

With swagger in our steps, and those of our trusted steed, we strode into Camp 3 just before the cutoff: Eco-Challenge 2019, 60 percent complete. Things were looking pretty good and I felt the rhythm and momentum. My TV interview at that checkpoint before heading back out on the course concluded on a positive note: "I'm confident that we'll finish the race."

TEN

Today is Thanksgiving. Let me be more precise:
today is the first Thanksgiving since my ALZ
diagnosis and the first Thanksgiving that I haven't
been entirely happy with everything in my life.

In our family, probably like most, at Thanksgiving
dinner we all sit around the table and recite what we
are thankful for. Of course this year, like every year,
I'm very thankful for Pammy and my kids and my
grandkids and everybody in the family. Right now,
however, as I sit in my office downstairs, I can't think
of anything I'm particularly thankful for this year.
In fact, the only thing I can think of at this point in
time is bullshit. Why did I have to get Alzheimer's
disease? Of course, we've been through that before
and there is no good answer. That is a bummer.

The good news is this year several of the family
members are out of town and won't arrive until
later tonight, and as a result we're going to have
our Thanksgiving on Friday, so I've got twenty-
four hours to think of something good to say. Or
maybe I'll snap out of this piss-poor attitude and
tell everybody how thankful I am that there is some
hope that my situation will improve dramatically
and I can return to a normal life without Alzheimer's
disease. I'll let you know how it turns out tomorrow.

—MACE'S JOURNAL
NOVEMBER 23, 2018

*I'm happy to say that the Thanksgiving dinner was
just about perfect. In fact, it was perfect. It was
great having all the grandkids, and my sister Boo
was there with her partner, Lynne, and of course,
my kids, Travis and Katelyn. We all had a great time
and I couldn't have asked for a better evening.*

—MACE'S JOURNAL
NOVEMBER 24, 2019

THE COLORADO AIR was hazy with wildfire smoke in
August 2020, but eleven months after Fiji, the route ahead
looked a bit clearer to the Macy family than it had prior to
Eco-Challenge. We were gathered at Mom and Dad's house
to watch the Amazon Prime debut of *World's Toughest Race:
Eco-Challenge Fiji 2019*. The wait had been long, and we
were pumped!

Amazon had told us that Team Endure would be one of
the featured teams and asked us to help promote the launch,
but that's about all we knew. With the COVID-19 pandemic
in full swing, binge-watching was in vogue, and we planned to
hammer through all ten episodes that day. It seemed like there
was a lot of online chatter about the series (at least in our little
adventure racing corner of the internet). Who knew, maybe
this series would be the next *Tiger King*? Probably not, but
we were excited anyway, particularly for my kids, Wyatt and
Lila, and nephew, Jaxon, to be able to see Grandpa in action
on TV, doing his thing. Those kids had been in Fiji, but only
back at the hotel after the race. Now, they'd really get to see
what the Eco-Challenge was about—and I'd need to explain
to them why we didn't finish the course, even though finishing
what you start is important and I had told the camera I was
confident we'd make it through.

Contemplating how to explain—in child-friendly terms—Alzheimer's and the race and why you should never quit until it's really time to quit, my mind drifted back to the months before Eco: the shock and sadness and frantic action following diagnosis; my own anxiety, depression, and panic about something so terrible and out of my control; the urgency to do something big and the uncertainty as we prepared for the race; the trials and joys of the race itself; and coming home to…what was it that I felt upon coming home?

Ease. Confidence. Acceptance.

Yes, after Eco-Challenge, I found myself handling the Alzheimer's journey a little better. Things weren't always bright (and I'm not telling you they are now, either), but going through the trenches in Fiji with Dad felt like a pivotal experience, a rite of passage. Sadness over the potential loss of Dad as my guide had become acceptance of my new role, a role that sons had taken on over generations and millennia. A role that I was now ready to embrace.

In my previous career as a high school English teacher, I worked with students to examine the archetypal hero's journey presented in many classic and contemporary texts, including various trials and tribulations that ultimately led to growth. In some courses I taught Dan Millman's *Way of the Peaceful Warrior*, and I appreciate what the author has said about the necessity of challenge before growth: "Every positive change—every jump to a higher level of energy and awareness—involves a rite of passage. Each time to ascend to a higher rung on the ladder of personal evolution, we must go through a period of discomfort, of initiation. I have never found an exception."

I thought also of my phone call with Ken Chlouber and Merilee Maupin, the longtime organizers of the Leadville Race Series. When I'd called them in early 2019 to tell them about Dad's diagnosis, Ken's response was crystal clear: "Well, son, it's time for you to step up and take the lead here." At the time, that had felt like a huge challenge that could only be overcome by a real hero, but now, after the Fijian rite of passage, it felt more like the natural course of life.

I'm not claiming to be any sort of hero, and the role I played in supporting my dad on the TV series simply portrays the courage and care that family members, friends, and community members exhibit every day in digging deep to support each other. That said, I do think there's value in cultivating and practicing our own "heroic mindsets"—and maybe even thinking through our own natural or constructed rites of passage.

(So, how can you think heroically as you navigate the challenges ahead, be they associated with Alzheimer's or something else? Are you going through something tough that could be reimagined as a rite of passage, including the possibility of some positive outcome? Is it time to construct an activity or challenge that represents a rite of passage for you, your family, your team, or your company?)

Back at my parents' house, I was now ready to discuss Alzheimer's with the kids in an appropriate manner— honest yet optimistic—without breaking down. I was ready to pause the show to answer their questions, laugh, and fill in the details. I knew they were going to see that Grandpa and I had set out confidently from Camp 3, only to return about ten hours later after deciding to stop racing because it was too dangerous and impossible to continue for us in those circumstances. Dad's back had deteriorated irreparably, and our progress in ascending a technical river canyon was very slow as we crisscrossed the increasingly violent, slippery, and rocky river dozens of times. Shane had remembered the upcoming canyoneering section well from the 2002 Eco-Challenge Fiji course: "We'll be swimming through long, deep pools of cold water and then scrambling to get back on top of the rocks and then swimming again. It's extremely cold up there." Swimming really would have been impossible at that point, and Shane summed up our situation: "Trav, I think we'd be walking ourselves into a rescue situation." Just then, a chopper cruised overhead. Dangling from it was a rescue bucket with a person in it, a person who had just been plucked off the course somewhere ahead. We came together as a team and made the safety-oriented decision that I then relayed to race director Kevin Hodder on our emergency radio: "Kev, it's Team Endure. We're turning around and heading back to Camp 3. Thanks for an incredible experience. And Dad's wondering if someone there has some IPAs for us!"

I stood by the decision and was absolutely at peace with it.

The kids would see us on TV as we staggered back to Camp 3 on our last legs, exhausted but ecstatic to hug our friends Bob, Marshall, Adrian, Heather, Andrew, and Nancy. The Stray Dogs had narrowly missed the Camp 3 cutoff that afternoon, and there we were, back together, to end it as one team. Marsh summed it up pretty well as Dad approached: "Man, you look like shit!" We all cracked up. The race was over for our teams, but we were happy, satisfied, and empowered to take on the uncertainty that lay ahead in real life as a team. Adventure races are tough, but you know that, one way or another, it'll all be over in a little more than a week. Life's real challenges—health, relationships, parenting, finances, whatever—don't have an end date or cutoff time, so we've got to be ready to keep hanging in there, doing our best alone and as a team, a mile at a time.

I also knew that when we watched the series, Dad's grandkids would remember something they experienced in Fiji but did not show up in the TV coverage: Dad receiving a new award called "The Spirit of Eco-Challenge" from Bear Grylls and the Eco producers. Bear's presentation of a fine, hand-crafted, small wooden camakau had the audience in tears, as did Dad's acceptance: "I gotta tell everyone here that the Eco-Challenge is an amazing event that has literally changed my life. I've done eight of these [applause], and it's all about the family."

We all had a blast watching the race. Dad and Mom laughed with the grandkids over stories about mud, huge bats, and Shane asking him, "Split a bar, Mace?" over and over. By the end of the day, even the inside of the house was hot and smoky from the wildfires across the West, but I'm proud to say we all made it through ten episodes in a single sitting (take that, *Tiger King*).

Shortly thereafter, Dad's newfound notoriety and recognizability out in the real world provided a nice boost and a bolstered platform that would enable him to spread the same message he'd been giving for years: "Do what you love. Keep the faith. Never quit." Passersby on the trails started to recognize Dad as "that Eco-Challenge guy." They'd say hello and ask how he was doing; he'd quickly shift the conversation to their own dreams, goals, and challenges, encouraging them to go big and stay positive. Dad's a natural coach and helper; encouraging others fulfills him, and I'm glad he continues to have opportunities to do it. Tech gets very challenging with Alzheimer's, and while Dad continues to enjoy scrolling Facebook, Mom and Katelyn have been very helpful in sharing his thoughts and stories via his Instagram account (@mmacy146), which grew exponentially after the race. Dad's schedule as a "retired old guy" has consistently included video calls with folks in the greater Alzheimer's community, including the Alzheimer's Association, support groups around the country, and other people with Alzheimer's and their families. Dad loves these calls, and I know his participation makes a big difference for people.

Looking back, it's clear that Alzheimer's forced us to accept the reality that many things in the world are much more uncertain and out of our control than we may have thought or wished. A few months after the race, the entire world was encountering some of the same realizations in addressing a shared challenge: COVID-19.

The pandemic was, and is as of this writing, a terrible event that can't be downplayed. That said, my parents' life was probably impacted even more by Alzheimer's. Mom is immunosuppressed due to her transplants and it's never good for someone with Alzheimer's to be hospitalized, so Mom and Dad had to be extremely careful. Family visits were very limited prevaccination, but they were thankful to live in a beautiful rural area where they could get outside daily for hikes, runs, and rides. The pandemic normalized video calls for work and family, and I like to think this may have allowed some Alzheimer's sufferers and caregivers to connect with family and friends more often than they had previously.

The proliferation of video calls also allowed Dad and me to engage in a new, shared professional project together: the Travis Macy Show Podcast (www.travismacy.com/podcast). I love talking with interesting people, and I had been thinking about starting a podcast for years by early 2021, when it dawned on me that this would be a great project to share with Dad. So, with the faith that things would work out if we worked hard and consistently, Dad and I began interviewing a new guest each week via recorded video call. We're almost a year in, and we've hit a stride, generating solid content with endurance athletes, authors, thought leaders, health experts, and more. Interpersonal communication remains one of Dad's strengths (in addition to fitness, relationships, camping, and encouraging others, to name a few more), and the guests and audience are always glad to hear from him. Yeah, there may be some repeated questions and trouble finding words from time to time, but who cares? In fact, I'm very proud to be part of a production that gives a public voice to someone going through Alzheimer's, and we hope this may be helpful in supporting others who don't want their voices to be silenced because of their so-called "limitations."

Shortly after Eco-Challenge, Dad and I started writing this book. I knew from experience that writing a book and getting it out there are much easier said than done, but we believed in the message and I was stoked to work with Dad. Plus, like adventure racing and life, book-writing is a team sport. We were lucky to work with our agent, Linda Konner, writers John Hanc and John Capouya, and later with writer Patrick Regan for the bulk of the text. Patrick became a close friend as we worked through the content and process, and we value his friendship and support. Writing has proven therapeutic and freeing for me, and I have been thoroughly impressed with Dad's perseverance in laboriously making his way through draft material, even while Alzheimer's makes it nearly impossible for him to read and write:

> *I feel like a fucking child. I used to be in charge*
> *of things. I was the one who decided what to*
> *do and how to do it and when to do it. Now I'm*
> *trying to read these emails about the book and I*
> *realize I'm behind the 8-ball; I can barely read*
> *this stuff and I certainly feel like I have no control*
> *about what's going on in this book process and*

everything else for that matter. The good thing is
I know I have good people taking care of me.

—Mace's Journal

Mom and Dad spent hours upon hours writing his journal material, him speaking while she transcribed. Dad was
for decades an avid reader of nonfiction, particularly history
and politics, and the loss of this element of his life saddens me
deeply. I know Dad's still a happy, resilient, and optimistic
person because he says so and acts as such, but it's hard to
live with the knowledge that some of his moments have felt
bleak.

In addition to the book and podcast, Dad has remained
active in the outdoors since Eco-Challenge. Cultivating
adventures along the lines of "as fast as we can, as slow as we
must," Dad gets after it outside every day. Technical mountain biking and exploring the woods on his own are activities
of the past, but at this point Dad can still bike and run alone
in the neighborhood on days when he doesn't go for a longer
trail run with me or friends like Marsh, Dr. Bob, Dean
Freeze, or Dale Peterson. Once those guys are out there,
they're just like any group of old dudes on the golf course or
in the coffee shop: just a bunch of big boys having fun, giving
each other shit, and laughing like crazy. So what if one guy
happens to have Alzheimer's? Everyone else has one issue or
another as well, and as a team they're a solid, committed unit.
The team commitment of Marsh and Heather Ulrich has
been particularly helpful and inspirational, and I'm always
grateful (not to mention impressed) when Marsh swings by
Dad's place to repair the snow blower or fix the woodpecker
holes in the house's siding. (Dad was never a mechanical
genius, and Alzheimer's hasn't exactly bolstered those skills.)

With most races canceled in 2020, Dad's summer focus was Leadville race series' Vertical Challenge, which pushed athletes to log as much "vert" as they could over eight weeks. Rather than logging mileage on the bike and foot, competitors tracked vertical gain. Hills have always been Dad's wheelhouse, so the two of us teamed up for the virtual event (meaning you could do it from wherever you happen to live). Dad has all day to train while I have kids and work, so I really had to push myself to keep up with his progress. Most days, he'd run in the morning, bike in the afternoon, and then hike laps up the hill behind the house, sometimes with Mom or the grandkids but more likely alone, keeping home in sight to avoid disorientation in the dusky woods. Dad often logged more than 3,000 feet of climbing in a day (in case that means nothing to you, well, it's a lot, especially at high altitude), and we each exceeded 100,000 feet of vert for the challenge. We each earned a Leadville buckle, and I'm still pumped about that for Dad.

After a bit of winter snowshoe racing, Dad's following spring and summer training and racing focused on a project with the Alzheimer's Association's The Longest Day. The association approached us about featuring Dad as a spokesperson to promote the fund-raiser, and he was all-in from the start. Heck, we were all all-in for this chance to support the Alzheimer's community and do something special alongside Dad.

The Alzheimer's Association's The Longest Day event is the largest annual fund-raiser for the country's most prominent Alzheimer's organization. It occurs on the longest day of the year, at the summer equinox, and is so named partly in commemoration of the long, long days that are spent by Alzheimer's caregivers. The association was very supportive in promoting Dad's story through its #BeLikeMace social media campaign.

The most significant and impactful single event of the Team Endure Longest Day fund-raiser was a project spearheaded by Marshall Ulrich and supported especially by Dr. Bob and Marsh's wife, Heather. For years, Marshall has been known as the "King of Death Valley," with dozens of crossings through America's hottest and lowest desert, both associated with the Badwater Ultramarathon and for his own journeys and FKTs.

In winter 2021, just months before his seventieth birthday, Marsh's latest big adventure was to trek across Death Valley and complete a winter mountaineering ascent of Mount Whitney in a first-ever running and mountaineering adventure he called Fire and Ice. After trekking all the way across Death Valley for 130+ miles on the road, Marsh met Dr. Bob and a climbing guide for a multiday winter mountaineering ascent of Mount Whitney, the highest peak in the lower forty-eight states. Meanwhile, Heather promoted the campaign through Facebook and other social media, raising over $15,000 for the Alzheimer's Association. Additional fundraising efforts spearheaded by Mom and supported by dozens of other friends and family members brought in another $15,000, bringing the total to more than $30,000.

Appropriately, The Longest Day fund-raiser culminated for our family on the longest day itself, June 21, in my new hometown of Salida, Colorado. We packed a lot in, including a 5k run; another short, steep running race up and down Tenderfoot Mountain, which sits just behind the historic downtown; and a 10k trail run that saw Dad and me traveling with an older woman who was running with an oxygen tank on her back as she rehabbed from her own cancer journey. We may have been at the back of the pack, but boy, did I feel proud to be out there with these two resilient people still doing their best at something they loved.

In addition to Dad's racing and daily exercise, I've been very impressed over the last couple of years with the resilient spirit displayed by Mom and Dad as they continue to embrace life fully each day—and that still includes travel. The old mantra applies: *as fast as we can, as slow as we must.* Maybe Mom and Dad can't travel anymore with the large travel trailer they dreamed of for years, but they're still getting out there, staying in rental homes and hotels, and even sleeping in a small conversion van they recently purchased. I always tell my coaching clients that *perfect is the enemy of good*, and Mom and Dad's resilience in pursuing their retirement dreams in the midst of significant adversity continues to prove that concept true for me. Traveling throughout Colorado, Mom and Dad often stop by to support my kids in their games and me in my races, including a new pursuit: pack burro racing, Colorado's official Heritage Sport, in which each trail runner travels with a donkey on a leash. Burro racing is a crazy adventure, and even though competing is no longer a good fit for Dad, we love being at the events together.

As evidenced by her years as an involved mother for her own kids and foster children, Mom is a caretaker at heart, but she's also self-aware and conscious of the importance of her own mental health and personal time. A few weeks ago, Mom was able to enjoy a trip with her girlfriends to see the fall colors of Colorado's Rocky Mountains. Although initially upset that he could not stay home alone and would instead need to stay with me and my family for the week, Dad was able to embrace that new reality and make the most of the time with our family, which we spent camping, running, hanging out around town, and watching the kids in their soccer and gymnastics practices. Again, things aren't perfect by any means, but we're all doing our best as a team to work through the day-to-day in a flexible and team-oriented manner.

In a final, optimistic note, just prior to this writing a new drug produced by Biogen called Aducanumab has been approved for limited use in treating early-stage Alzheimer's. The drug has come to market amidst some skepticism and uncertainty, but I personally see the approval as a very positive step because it's the first medication targeted toward treating the root causes of Alzheimer's rather than merely mitigating symptoms. We've explored the drug with multiple neurologists, and it seems that unfortunately Dad's disease course has probably moved beyond the relevance of this particular medication, but I'm optimistic that it may be able to help others now and in the future, in addition to paving the way for other similar medications that may be used much earlier in the disease progression.

For years, it's been commonplace for people in their twenties, thirties, and forties to receive cholesterol tests, and if things are not looking good on the track to, say, coronary artery disease, they may begin a drug treatment that keeps things from getting bad before a full-on disease process has even begun. Similarly, I hope that those who are concerned about Alzheimer's, including myself and many other children and grandchildren of people who have been diagnosed with a disease, may be able to undergo routine tests for plaques and tangles in the brain and then intervene with medications that stop things from getting bad well before a disease would have been diagnosed. For those reading who may be concerned about their own cognitive decline, be it imminent or hypothetical and futuristic like my own personal concerns, I want to tell you that I know your anxiety can be significant and real as it has been for me since my dad was diagnosed. I want you to know that you're not in this alone, that we can all be a team as we move through life together, and that there are lots of smart people putting a lot of work into medical treatments and tests that may be able to help us. Also, for what it's worth, since Dad was diagnosed I've personally put much greater emphasis on my own sleep and healthy eating as I know these are absolutely imperative to brain health. Whereas in the past not needing sleep was often seen as a badge of honor, particularly for goal-driven, type A men like me who like to work hard, exercise hard, and play hard, it's now becoming more accepted that, even if we don't like it, we're all just humans and we all need to practice consistent, solid sleep habits.

For detailed information on nutrition as related to cognition, please explore www.brainhealthkitchen.com.

ELEVEN

I guess there's only one thing to do at a time like this. More miles.

—MACE'S JOURNAL
OCTOBER 16, 2021

ACCEPTANCE IS NOT A DESTINATION, not a static state. Three years ago today, we received Dad's diagnosis. And here we are still treading water in a sea of ambiguous loss. In that span, unexpected things have happened. His cognitive decline has progressed more slowly than most would have guessed—certainly slower than anticipated by the neurologist who, after submitting Dad to a series of tests back in the fall of 2018, urged him to get his affairs in order, seriously pissing him off in the process.

Three years is a long time. As much as any of us hated the idea of Dad with Alzheimer's being the new normal, well, it's kind of unavoidable after three years. Some days—sometimes for a span of days—Dad seems to accept this condition—accept that he can't change it and therefore must make the best of it—whatever that looks like. Other days, he's just as pissed off as he was at that neurologist three years ago. There is no cure for Alzheimer's. There is no proven treatment. But there is therapy. For Dad—and for me, too—that therapy is to run.

Since I was a little kid, Dad and I have run up mountains together. Big mountains. The first 14,000-footer we ever ran up together was Grays Peak. I was thirteen years old. I

200

remember how we'd run together on the trail for a time, until Dad would slowly pull away, and in doing so, pull me along the trail after him. *"Keep hammerin', Bud!"* Was he saying those words for the millionth time or was I just hearing them echo? It didn't matter. Their origin was as clear as their message. *"You can do this. You can beat this. You're stronger than you know."* At the summit, I'd find him sitting on a rock, waiting for me. He'd stand up, put his arm around me, and lean in close so his head was touching mine, just as he always did. "Way to hammer, Bud. I'm proud of you." Another peak conquered, and another magical day on the trail with Dad.

With each passing month, I had less trouble keeping up with Dad on the trail. Our strides were different—he's more long-legged than I—but for a brief window in time, our pace matched up. And then I started pulling away from him on the ascents, and he'd find me waiting for him at the summit. How many miles? How many footfalls? How many heart-beats shared on these mountain trails? And how many more to come?

A few months ago, Dad and I went back to Leadville. Not for the 100 this time, but for the Silver Rush 50. Dad hadn't run a race this long in years, and in fact he hadn't run a Leadville ultra since 1995, though he was certainly capable.

It's not completely accurate to say he hadn't run in Leadville since 1995, though. In truth, he'd probably run the equivalent of several 100-milers on the Leadville courses since the last time he was officially entered. Dad hasn't been competing in the Leadville ultras, but he's been assisting other racers—family members, friends, sometimes even strangers—by serving as pacer. If you're not part of the long-distance running community, you may not be familiar with the term. The natural assumption would be that a pacer helps a runner to maintain a certain pace in a race, and in a broad sense that's true, but pacing someone involves a lot more, and it requires a certain skill set and spirit that Dad wholly embodies.

First, of course, a pacer must be able to run as fast as the runner he or she is pacing—at least for the part of the course the pacer is pacing. You certainly don't want to slow your runner down. But being able to run with someone stride for stride for a few (or several) miles is just the beginning. As a pacer, your job, at various points in a race, may be to provide emotional support, assess physical and mental state, distract from minor (or not-so-minor) aches and pains, encourage nutrition and hydration (like Shane force-feeding me Cheetos during my 2013 Leadman run), sing *Eye of the Tiger*... essentially provide whatever your runner needs and remove as many barriers to success as you can. After running thirty or fifty or even ninety-nine miles, a runner isn't necessarily thinking perfectly straight. A pacer provides clear-eyed decision making. Drink this. Eat this. Get ready for the climb ahead. So, pacing isn't really about setting a pace. It's about *getting a runner through,* even when—especially when— that runner loses confidence in himself or herself. It's about keeping them from giving up. Over the past quarter of a century, I doubt that anyone has served as a more frequent or effective pacer than my dad. He's not just good at it—he loves to do it. In fact, he'll tell you that he likes pacing way more than racing. Even more than his multiple 100-mile finishes, I'd say that Dad's true Leadville legacy is all the people he's helped get across the finish line.

Dad, naturally, brushes off these efforts as no big deal. "You just putz along with someone and bullshit and make sure they're okay," he says. "It's a lot of fun."

Fun was definitely what Dad brought to the table when he paced his Stray Dogs teammate, Dr. Bob Haugh, in the second half of the Leadville 100 in 2005. Bob was a veteran endurance athlete with a couple of 100-milers under his belt by then, but none at 10,000+ feet. (Bob's hometown of Paducah, KY, sits at about 400 feet above sea level.) Bob actually had more company than just Dad on this run. Marshall Ulrich ran most of the race with him, and I also joined in for the last twenty-five miles or so. For Dr. Bob, Dad's pacing amounted mostly to keeping him amusingly distracted by unspooling stories about past adventure races they'd done together.

"We told the same stories we've told twenty times before," Bob remembers, "'You remember that time we were out on the kayaks and the storm came? And I was scared shit-less and you were scared shitless... yeah, yeah, yeah!' Those same old stories kept me going and kept me laughing.... Mark and I were yukking it up so much that Marshall was getting aggravated with us because he was afraid we were going to miss the cutoff time." No worries. The pace was perfect, and Dr. Bob finished with twenty minutes to spare.

The night after the race, Dr. Bob recalls needing to crawl across his hotel room to answer the phone. He was in too much pain to stand. But out on the course, the lively conversation with his wisecracking buddy had kept pain and despair at bay. "We just traipsed along in the middle of the night having a grand time. For most people, they're just in total agony by mile 75 or 80. We all had a great time, and saying that about the Leadville 100, you know, that's really saying something." It certainly is. In all my years of being around the Leadville races and racers, I've *never* heard anyone say they "just traipsed along." Gotta love Dr. Bob.

We all have our favorite pacing stories involving Dad, but one of the all-time classics—and one that speaks volumes about Dad—involves his brother-in-law, my uncle Tim. Tim had entered the Leadville 100 in 2003 but exited with a disappointing

DNF (did not finish) next to his name. When he decided to try again, Dad was determined to get Tim in under the thirty-hour cutoff and get him that finisher's buckle. As he had with Dr. Bob the year before, Dad would pace Tim for the final fifty miles of the race.

There's no source like a primary source, so I'm going to let Uncle Tim tell this story:

Mace and I both have intense lower back pain issues when we run long distances, always have. Accordingly, I was experiencing extreme back pain during the run from May Queen at mile 87.5 and stopped every half mile to bend over and stretch my back. Mace kept saying, "Tim, I know that feels good, [being simultaneously empathetic and sympathetic] but you will never finish if you keep doing that." Mace was "nurturing" but increasingly frustrated, which engendered the "you will never finish" coda.

As we were running the last six miles to the finish line—what's commonly known as "the Boulevard," we encountered more than forty racers who were walking, quite certain they had the finish "in the bag." Mace started telling them that they would not finish if they kept walking. So now Mace is pacing me and forty other runners. This was fine with me because Mace had already set me up for a last-minute finish, and I respected what he was doing for all these other runners he had never met. He truly wanted them to finish because he knew how important finishing is at Leadville...or at anything in life, which is what he is all about. He made it his purpose to help get them to the finish line in under thirty hours. You have to finish it, get it done. You just have to.

One among the pack of forty runners was a German guy, great guy, but he was depleted and walking with the pack of runners destined to not finish. He listened and respected Mace's warning and suddenly split from the pack and joined Mace and me. We ran all the way in and he let me finish a couple of minutes before him, which is Leadville protocol, but also in deference to his new mentor, Mace. Little did he know that he and I had the same mentor. I'll never be able to express my appreciation for what Mace did for me that day. I've tried, and he characteristically won't accept it, but I know he did more for me and that other runner than he'll ever know. To me, this is the story of Mace: selfless, caring, and willing do anything to help someone else achieve a significant goal that matters to them.

Uncle Tim recently found himself in an even bigger battle, one with cancer. Just as at Leadville, he's taken it step by step, as fast as he can, as slow as he must. He's winning the race and things are looking good; I have no doubt the mental training from Leadville has been an asset on this journey.

Following Dad's example, I've helped pace for some of the top endurance athletes of my generation. One of my most memorable experiences was pacing Emma Roca (yup, the same Emma from Eco-Challenge in Fiji) in 2014, the year after I won Leadman.

Emma had come all the way from Catalonia and was gunning for a win (as she usually was) in the LT100, and I signed on to pace her for the final twenty-six miles of the race. I wrote about the race—definitely a learning experience for me—in *Ultrarunning* magazine:

Things started smooth enough when I joined Emma at dusk. She had been in second place all day, and we both felt good as we travelled together over all of those false summits on Powerline. I thought about Emma's pace, her mindset, her caloric intake and hydration, her clothing needs and lighting options. I reminded her to eat and drink, talked about the course to come, and offered my best cheerleading on staying positive and believing a come-from-behind win was possible.

And, before we knew it, the win really was possible.

Emma took the lead with 10 miles to go! She was feeling great and psyched to hammer it in along what my dad lovingly calls "the longest lake in the world" (if you've done Leadville, you know he's right).

One problem: Two minutes after Emma took the lead, I was on the side of the trail puking my guts out!

Emma wasn't waiting for me, and rightly so— she had a race to win. And I knew I had to get my act together. I finished barfing, chased hard and made the catch, ran for a few minutes, and ralfed again. After a number of cycles of this nonsense,

I realized my thinking process needed to change ASAP if I was going to help Emma win the race.

When we suffer on race day (or pace day), the natural inclination is to think about what we are doing: the pain of each step, the nauseous pressure in the gut, blisters growing and growing. What we should do, however, when the going gets tough, is think about why we are doing it: the achievement, the glory, the experience, lessons for our kids, social media posts, water cooler bragging rights... whatever!

There is a time to think about what you are doing. Wise runners pay attention early in the race to pace and feel and fuel rather than dreaming of glory. As we saw, I spent most of my first fifteen miles of pacing thinking about Emma's needs. That's great—except that I completely neglected my own nutrition and hydration, resulting in the puke-fest down the road.

Lesson learned: When doing something detail-oriented (like making sure you eat, drink, and pace correctly, especially early in a race) think about what you are doing. Later, when you enter the pain cave, think why.

I shifted my thinking out there with Emma, and I'm happy to say we made it up the Boulevard together for the win.

I'll never forget my introduction to Emma. During an adventure race through a Mexican desert in 2005, I pushed my bike up a steep hill with teammates Dave Mackey and Danelle Ballengee. We were all strong athletes, but we were barely making it up this thing. Out of nowhere, a female racer approached from behind, carrying a bike on her shoulders as she strode past us at a quick pace and then moved ahead, out of sight. Shortly thereafter, she came running back down the hill without the bike; we could now see she was the feared competitor Emma Roca, known well on the circuit as the bulletproof captain of Spain's Team Buff. Some time later, Emma returned from behind, towing her male teammate on a bungee cord while carrying his bike as they passed us again.

Emma's strength and endurance became legendary in adventure racing as she led her team to the world championship in 2010 before shifting focus to ultrarunning so she could spend more time with her kids and bring them overseas for extended summer trips of racing and travel. She finished 3rd at Ultra Trail du Mont Blanc (UTMB) in 2012 and 2013 and then focused on events in the US: Run Rabbit Run (1st, 2nd, 2nd); Leadville (1st); Hardrock (2nd); and Western States (5th). Emma was clearly at these races to compete, but the summer trips were all about family and friends as she shared her knowledge, company, and contagious enthusiasm with many of us around the country who were fortunate enough to befriend her. We trained together, discussing life, culture, and exercise science; shared kids' birthdays with vibrant, multilingual parties; supported her husband, David, when he mountain-biked the Colorado Trail; and relaxed on river-rafting trips, enjoying the Colorado sun and views. It seemed the good times with Emma and her family would go on for decades—we probably didn't know how good we had it.

Events like life-threatening liver disease, Alzheimer's, and the early death of a good person force people to grapple with big questions. Why me (or him or her)? Why now? How could a benevolent higher power allow this to happen? How can I handle this and be happy again?

My opinion: we're all entitled to our own conclusions, and none is better than any other. If it works for you, then keep believing it. For me, life is certainly biological, partially spiritual, tenuous always, wonderful hopefully, painful sometimes, generally uncertain. Make the most of it. Every. Single. Day. Focus on the present, but keep the long view and be patient.

Pain and uncertainty came quickly to the forefront when Emma Roca—vibrant, energetic, optimistic Emma from Eco-Challenge and Leadville, who inspired thousands and seemed a big sister to me—told us of her cancer diagnosis in 2020.

Emma began seeing gynecologists in January 2020. Misdiagnoses and COVID-related delays preceded a summer diagnosis of vulvar carcinoma. Radiation, chemotherapy, and a vulvectomy had Emma feeling strong and all of us optimistic as of February 2021; she even told me of her plans to write an informative and empowering book on this uncommon type of cancer. But things quickly turned for the worse when the cancer went systemic.

A few years earlier I had been pacing Emma in the Hardrock 100, one of the toughest ultras anywhere. Deep in the night and high in the mountains, we fell into an ice-cold beaver pond that had encroached on the trail. We were both dangerously cold, especially Emma because she'd been going for eighty miles. We kept our heads, helped each other into dry clothes, rejuvenated with warm hot chocolate and crunchy bacon at the next aid station, and were rewarded with a rare and magical lynx sighting at sunrise and Emma's second-place finish a few hours later. I supported Emma at Hardrock and she supported Dad and me with tears and hugs as we embraced before and after Eco-Challenge in Fiji. Her encouragement and teamwork empowered my Alzheimer's journey.

In some bleak situations, calm teamwork, smooth level-headedness, and bold optimism save the day.

This cancer deal wasn't one of those situations.

Would I have done or said anything different in Fiji if I'd known I would never see Emma again? I rarely said "I love you" to Dad for years because it didn't seem manly and I knew he knew, but now I say it all the time. Did Emma know how much I admired her and appreciated her friendship? I told her as much on many video calls over those months of decline, and I scrambled to get to Barcelona as things looked bad, but COVID prevented the travel.

Emma Roca of Catalonia—wife of David and mother of Irina, Marti, and Mariona and friend of hundreds—passed away on June 18, 2021, at age forty-seven.

If a lifetime can be judged by the positive impact it leaves on those who live on, then Emma's is just as she was on the racecourse: one in a million. We love you, Emma, and we'll never forget you.

I think of Emma every day when I look up at the Angel of Shavano, an ever-present snow feature on a high peak that I can see from home. Like my memories of Emma, it's a happy spot, and one she would have loved. I'm trying to be at peace with sadness and a simultaneous optimism (like Emma's), alongside angry disillusionment about bullshit stories like, "Everything happens for a reason," which some people use to explain away occurrences like untimely death and Alzheimer's.

Man, this life stuff is some strong shit. I need to go for a run.

I think I said something before about *ease* and *acceptance*, so back to the summer of 2021 and the Silver Rush 50. Dad and

I would run this one together, something we'd never done before. As I'd learned in Fiji, supporting an athlete with Alzheimer's involves different types of care and a deeper level of forethought. But at least we wouldn't be slogging through a muddy jungle or paddling a wobbly homemade kayak. We'd be running on a bright summer day on a course that both of us knew like it was our backyard—which, in a sense, it was. Running in Leadville always made us feel like we had home-field advantage.

In many ways, Dad is old-school on the trail. He never saw much need to explore or embrace the science of nutrition, hydration, calorie burn rates, heart-rate monitoring, and the like. I, however, took all that into account when planning our Silver Rush 50 run in 2021.

As is our usual race weekend tradition, we camped the night before at the Sugar Loafin' campground just outside of Leadville, and we were up early to make the 6:00 a.m. start. At 10,000 feet altitude even mid-July mornings can be nippy, and this one was in the thirties. Still, our spirits were nothing but warm as we enjoyed a prerace powwow with old friends and race cofounders Ken Chlouber and Merilee Maupin. It was a true family affair, as our circle of supporters also included Ken's son, Cole; Mom and Amy and our kids, Wyatt and Lila; and my sister's family.

Making our final preparations, I offered Dad some sunscreen. "I've got Alzheimer's, Bud! You think I give a shit about skin cancer?!" We all cracked up. Even at this uncertain stage, Dad was still ready to crack a joke before running fifty miles at 10,000 feet. The gun went off and we eased into the day, hiking slowly up Dutch Henry Hill (used for skiing and sledding a few months later) with Wyatt, Lila, and Jaxon. The grandkids could sense Dad's pseudoroyalty status in this crowd, and they were totally pumped to partake for a few minutes.

Once the sun peeked over the mountains, the day began to warm, and Dad and I were feeling great as we knocked off the miles. Because of COVID-19 cancellations the previous year, this was the first big race Dad had been in since the World's Toughest Race in Fiji, and his celebrity status was obvious. Throughout the day, race fans and fellow runners shouted encouragement—even if they only knew it was "that guy from the Eco-Challenge." Dad loved the attention and stopped several times to pose for pictures. I knew that we didn't have a lot of time to spare as our eighteen-minutes-per-mile average speed would leave a razor-thin margin to make the twenty-five-mile cutoff, but, honestly, I didn't care. Dad was in his element. We were running together in the thin air on a gorgeous summer day being cheered on by the people we loved most in the world—and by friendly strangers too!

That thin air, in fact, was one of my primary worries leading up to that day—not for the lack of oxygen (we were used to that) but for the high level of particulates, courtesy of the wildland fires raging throughout the West. The Colorado Department of Public Health and Environment had issued air quality alerts every day for the preceding two weeks in Denver and other front-range cities and cautioned against outdoor recreation. I fretted a bit about running fifty miles in such conditions, but as it turned out, air quality at two miles high was significantly better than in the Mile High City and we were able to run with no respiratory problems.

We made the twenty-five-mile cutoff with a few minutes to spare. At the aid station, we enjoyed high fives and hugs from our support crew, grabbed a snack, and were off again. I knew the odds were against us making the next cutoff at mile 32, and I let Dad know that we might be timed out. Our pace remained steady. We passed runners on the climbs, and the same runners would pass us on the descents. Dad is still a racer at heart, and as much as he exhibits a laid-back air, he's more competitive than he lets on. But just as in Fiji, Dad's illusory perception of the downhill slopes kept him tentative. *As fast as we can... as slow as we must.* Marshall joined us for several miles that afternoon; the team was back together again, and there were Heather and Dr. Bob at an aid station to support with food and water—and more importantly with smiles and encouragement.

Most of the Silver Rush is run on dirt roads, and a few miles from the 32-mile aid station, a race support truck ("sag wagon") pulled alongside us. The driver asked if we wanted to ride the rest of the way. The race crew had obviously done the math as I had and knew that our day was coming to an end. I looked over at Dad but knew what was coming. "Hell no, we don't want a ride!" he said. On we ran. I'd been using my phone to check in with Mom along the way, and she had already talked to Uncle Eric, who would meet us at the 32-mile checkpoint. When we arrived there, missing the nine-hour cutoff by about thirty minutes, volunteers were busy packing up the aid station, but Eric was there with ice cream bars and cold Cokes. Dad was disappointed to miss the cutoff but happy to have had "the full experience." After all, we had been out on the course much longer than the winners, so I'd say we got our money's worth! As for me, I was just damn proud of Dad. To keep things in perspective, he had just run thirty-two miles at 10,000 feet in nine and a half hours at age sixty-eight with Alzheimer's. So, yeah, I'd call that a pretty good day.

The aspen leaves have fallen and another Rocky Mountain winter looms. As I finish this book, I find my mind returning often to our nine and a half hours on the trail last July. Should I ever suffer the ravages of a disease that steals away memories, let me please retain the images of that golden summer day with Dad. The trail-racing season is pretty much over now in our part of the country, but I've been thinking a lot lately about the whole notion of "pacing." Will I pace Dad again in a trail race, in Leadville or anywhere, next year? I would certainly never doubt him, but it all depends on the insidious progression of his disease (not to mention this nagging pandemic that continues to cancel many events). In Alzheimer's as in life, Managing Uncertainty is the name of the game.

What I do know is that for Mom, Katelyn, Dona, and me, and the rest of our family and friends, our role in "pacing" Dad is only beginning. As his mind falters, we will be there to guide his steps and buoy his spirit so it keeps soaring. When he perceives new dangers in the familiar world around him, we will calm him. When confusion reigns and frustrations build, we will clasp his hand and lead him through the darkness. In any ultradistance race, there comes a point where every step becomes a battle. Our job now is to help Dad take those steps and cover the distance that still lies between him and the finish line, no matter how far that may be. A mile at a time.

EPILOGUE

IN RACING PARLANCE, DNF stands for Did Not Finish. It is short for disappointment. An ignominious exit. Failure. It's what every athlete dreads seeing next to his or her name where a finishing time should be.

DNF is a final accounting merciless in its concision. It doesn't bother to take into account the myriad possible reasons why a competitor's race may have ended early—injury, illness, accident, utter exhaustion, or even failure to make a preordained cutoff time. I'd like to take back these potent little letters and recast them as something other than shorthand for failure, to remove their sting and their stigma.

Throughout his career and his life, Dad prided himself on seeing things through—on finishing. It's a lesson he learned from his own dad and imparted to me. I know that it crushed him and he blamed himself that our team had to pull out of Eco-Challenge Fiji after seven days, and it likewise bugged the hell out of him to miss the cutoff 32 miles into the 50-mile Silver Rush race in the summer of 2021. His last two major races resulted in something very rare in his nearly forty years of racing: a DNF next to his name.

I just can't leave it at that. I was with Dad for every step of both of those races. I can tell you that he never, ever quit. Not on the race, not on the team, not on himself. Sometimes, it's just out of your control. A lesson for racing and for living.

I felt compelled to add this epilogue because I want to make that distinction for Dad, but mostly because I want to suggest to the reader that despite traditional wisdom, finishing is actually the least important of the three parts of the race that is life.

Dad always joked that he won a lot of masters snowshoe races because he was the only one his age who showed up. "You beat all the people too scared to do it," he'd say with a glint in his eyes. There was playfulness in those blue eyes, but steeliness too. It's not *how* you start, but *that* you start.

The way you run—or swim or ride or work or love or parent or play—is even more important. How do you approach the challenge? How do you push yourself? How much do you believe? How deeply do you feel? How much are you willing to give? That, in essence, is what this contest—life—is all about. The end—the finish—will come for us all. The time stamp or the letters after your name will ultimately mean nothing. How you lived your life, what you put into it, and that you had the courage to truly show up for it in the first place—that is what counts. Do Not Forget that, or, to be concise: DNF.

DON'T TURN OUT THE LIGHTS ON LIFE

Milestones from Our
Alzheimer's Journey that Might
Help You Find Your Way, Too

HERE ARE SOME PRINCIPLES and actionable advice the Macy family and I developed on our Alzheimer's journey, to help you thrive when facing that or other major challenges and uncertainties. My hope is that they inspire you, too. Whether the distress is yours or a loved one's, try these tools and tactics. See what works for you.

—TRAVIS MACY

Bula! What We Can Learn from Rural Fijians
During the Eco-Challenge in Fiji you've just read about, Dad and I took a lot of positives from wonderful people who live simply:

Slow down. Appreciate being. Be present. Value family time. Live communally. Help each other. Be active. Exist in nature. Radiate enthusiasm. Go outside. Celebrate often. Eat together. Grow food. Give generously. Accept unconditionally. Dress vibrantly. Smile always.

Life Is a Team Sport, and You Get to Pick Your Team
While we've got to be bold in the face of adversity, we must also be humble in realizing we all need help. You can—and will—lead a team of family, friends, and medical professionals. You're a leader, yet you also need help; that's

okay and it's part of the deal. Proactively select your team, considering both capability and attitude.

Maybe there's some relief in talking with the friend who typically pulls you into bitching about the situation, but might it be more productive to spend more time with the other friend who sympathizes but also tends to help you stay positive, believe in yourself, and think creatively? If the doc you've been working with seems burned out and impersonal—maybe it's time to cut him or her loose and try a new draft pick. You can't choose your family members, but you do have a choice about which ones you'll talk with most, and a chance to set a contagious tone and attitude that may even rub off on some of the more difficult ones.

Bad Stories, Good Stories: The Ones You Tell Yourself Make All the Difference (Revisited)

Of all the principles from my first book, *The Ultra Mindset*, this one is not only the most relevant to Alzheimer's and other types of uncertainty but also the toughest one for me to master. Maybe you're like me in that your mind tends to cling tightly to certain ideas. This is great when the vibes are moving in the right direction, but it can make things go south quickly when the story turns negative. By gaining some distance on our thoughts and stories and seeing that they are just that—thoughts and stories, not *the truth*—we are more likely to realize the power to change them if needed. I often tell myself, I don't have to believe everything I think.

Try using the "good story" mindset to rewrite a deficit-focused story about yourself or someone else, so it shifts focus to one or more strengths. Dad's "I can't even drive myself to the trailhead anymore" becomes "I still enjoy running the trail at Evergreen Mountain after my wife drops me off there." Similarly, "I can't even travel in an airplane alone" shifts to "I enjoy the view from the passenger seat while taking road trips with Travis and Wyatt in my old truck."

For the caregiver, "I'm stuck at home doing this all day" might shift to something like "I can show her how much I still value our marriage by continuing to support her while also asking for the help from others that gives me some time for myself."

Rewriting stories never really ends, and on the Alzheimer's journey the same story will probably need to be revised many times as capabilities shift. I keep my most important good stories in a calendar item on my phone that I read each morning while waking up with a yoga routine. One example: "Depression and anxiety and anger may get seats in the car, but they don't get to drive."

Ambiguous Loss 101: It's OK to Cry during Country Songs

In an "ambiguous loss," one that has an uncertain scope and sequence like Alzheimer's, we've got to expect cycles of grief—but not necessarily the predictable stages we've all heard of, such as anger, denial, etc., that can follow a more finite, absolute loss, like the death of a family member. During these losses without closure things will feel stable at times. At other times the sadness or anger or sense of being overwhelmed will be just below the surface. We might feel like we're trucking along just fine until we hear country music lyrics like "I drive your truck" or "Love without end, amen." At that point we lose it and break into tears, or I do, for sure. And that's okay. That's release, catharsis—and it's why everyone should listen to country music.

The Wilderness Doesn't Give a Shit: Use Nature to Make Yourself (and Your Problems) Smaller and Appreciate Inevitable Cycles

Nature doesn't care who you are; experience (or lack thereof) and diagnosis (or lack thereof) are irrelevant in the woods. For people who face hourly reminders of their disabilities in the urban world of numbers, letters, details, and constant judgment, the wilderness can provide an empowering safe haven. Dad can't balance a checkbook anymore, but while hiking or running the Colorado mountains he's in his element, proficient and at ease. Nature's vastness—the stars in the sky free of light pollution or the endless emptiness of the rolling plains—reminds us that, in the scheme of things and history of humanity, our individual challenges aren't really that big.

Experiencing natural cycles like the salmon run, the Alaskan tides, or the annual growth of elk antlers before their owner is harvested and then brought to table reminds us that human cycles like aging and role-changing are natural and unavoidable.

Level the Playing Field

Maybe the wilderness isn't your thing, and that's just fine. The point is this: Use creativity to level the playing field for yourself or someone with Alzheimer's by searching out environments where deficits are minimized. Maybe Nana can't teach calculus anymore, but I bet she could have a lot of fun—and help out some teachers—volunteering at a local daycare while you enjoy some exercise or work time. Uncle Rob can't get to the tennis court or call out confusing scores like "thirty-love" anymore, but I bet he would love it if you could get one or two of his buddies to come over for some ping-pong, which requires less mobility and even uses regular numbers for scorekeeping.

The What's Next? Mindset: Staying Engaged by Keeping Something Big around the Corner.

Make sure you and your loved one always have something big coming up. "Something big" may evolve from taking on a 400-mile Eco-Challenge to a camping trip to a short hike. "Active travel" may shift from a self-guided international expedition to a cruise to a local road trip to visiting the grandkids to watching the Travel Channel. Even if "intellectual stimulation" used to mean rocket science, there may be a point when reading to a young child is just as fulfilling (and challenging). Whether you have a diagnosis or not, take time to make plans for things that keep you stoked on life.

"This Is Bullshit!": Accept and Fight

Tough diagnoses force us to embrace nuance, uncertainty, and ambiguity. Push yourself to accept the current reality while still fighting against limitations, naysayers, and societal assumptions and judgments. Embracing opposing truths simultaneously proves important with Alzheimer's because we must stay present with current strengths while also glancing to the future and planning responsibly.

The Swampland of Despair Sucks. And It Forces You to (Finally) Grow Up.

As all of us who've lived through the pandemic know, we can't help but be changed by prolonged entanglement with vast and uncertain challenges. As you change, approach the new you with curiosity. Might your own low moments allow you to be more empathetic with others when they struggle? Have you taken research professor Brene Brown's advice and moved from a story like *People need to pull up their bootstraps and take care of themselves* toward *Most people are truly doing their best most of the time; we all must be ready to generously give and accept help*? Psychologist Carl Jung's "two halves of life" presents a framework for growth through adversity as we move from a "first half" that's more focused on self and ego to a "second half" in which ego is less important and we can really focus on our meaningful, authentic contributions to the world.

Find Viktor Frankl's Space: Recognize Your Habits to Increase Control over Response

Holocaust survivor, psychiatrist, and neurologist Viktor Frankl was right: "Between stimulus and response there is a space. In that space is our power to choose our response. In our response lies our growth and our freedom."

Taking stock of our generalized and acute triggers and the responses that follow empowers us to change (if needed), grow (whether we want to or not), and (most importantly) rewrite our internal narratives so that we may move from despair to focusing on strengths.

Personally, when I am triggered by, say, the challenging marital conversations that are inherently part of the contract, I find that pausing to literally embrace the "space" with a little exercise or walk with the dogs or talk with my therapist helps me move toward a response that's less combative and more loving. Similarly, a caregiver who is triggered by an accident or mess or medical news in an already overwhelming environment might be able to use the space to choose what's immediately important, what can wait, and what is beyond their control—and then respond with thoughtful intention instead of knee-jerk reaction.

Professor Horton Says: "It Never Always Gets Worse."

An ultrarunning college professor (he actually had the students run a 50k for the final exam in one course) named David Horton gave that advice in a lecture I attended, and it really stuck with me. Dr. Horton seemed to be talking about running *and* about life: sometimes all data suggests that things can't possibly get any better... but then they do. Many nights in adventure races, struggling to stay awake until the damn sun finally comes up, I've sung along in my head with the Mamas and the Papas: "The darkest hour is just before dawn." (That's from "Dedicated to the One I Love"—not a country song but still good).

The Alzheimer's journey will probably go through some bleak territory. But, if we hang in there and "keep the faith" as Dad often recommends, there's a chance that things might get better. For Dad and me, acceptance has increased and anger has decreased a couple of years after diagnosis. Many people with ALZ have especially bad days and especially good days. If someone with ALZ gets sick (say, a urinary tract infection), cognition can go way down—and then often go back up if that temporary illness is resolved. While some ALZ patients experience negative personality shifts, some experience positive shifts. Depending on your spiritual preferences, you might "keep the faith" in a higher power or simply in yourself and your resilience.

As Fast as We Can, as Slow as We Must

Use nuanced thinking and planning to keep living fully, moving as fast as you can. At the same time, slow down and modify activities, commitments, and engagements, embracing empathy for you and yours as you progress as slow as you must. Maybe Mace can't run a hundred miles anymore, but he can probably manage a 50k. Maybe grandpa can't go on a backpacking mountain hunt due to his heart condition, but I bet he could take Billy duck hunting. Auntie might not be able to attend the weeklong craft fair to sell the chairs she makes because her immune system is so weak, but I bet you could help her invite some younger women to her apartment so she can teach them the skills she has mastered over the decades. Don't turn out the lights on life; keep living fully (and slowly shifting what that means).

Tip from the Top (10,200 Feet High, to Be Precise): "You're Better than You Think You Are. You Can Do More than You Think You Can."

Each year before an epic ride or run of a hundred miles in the Rocky Mountains, longtime Leadville 100 race director Ken Chlouber spoke these words to me, Dad, and everyone else packed into Leadville's 6th Street Gym at 10,200 feet. Ken was right that endurance competitions push us to do more than we think is possible. And he was even more right in suggesting that "you can do more than you think you can" in life beyond the racecourse, especially when it comes to supporting family. When Dad was diagnosed with ALZ, I called Ken and Merilee Maupin, his partner in race directing and life. Though saddened, they were clear: "Son, it's time for you to dig deep and step up and support your family here."

Ken and Merilee were right, and now I'm telling you to do the same.

A VOICE FOR THE VOICELESS

Alzheimer's patient Mark Macy's advice on how to treat the loved one in your life battling ALZ

Don't define me by my Alzheimer's

Since my diagnosis three years ago, I have been trying to continue my life as it has always been. In my case, since I've been involved in endurance sports for almost forty years, it's vital for me that I keep on running, hiking, and bicycling. Maybe not as fast or as far, but trying to get outside most days—even if it's just for a run through the trails behind my house in Evergreen, Colorado—is absolutely critical for my mental and physical well-being.

For other people, of course, it might be something different: music, art, a hobby. Whatever it is they love to do, it's important that they be encouraged and allowed to keep doing that, to the best of their ability. Continuing to enjoy that passion will keep your loved one anchored to his or her identity, and thus will keep them in your life as the person you know and love just a little bit longer. Stay engaged.

Stay connected with the world around you

For most of my life, I've tried to keep up with what's going on in the world. As an attorney, my day started with a thorough read of the *Wall Street Journal*. At night, I'd always try to make time for reading, often books about history.

It's hard for me now to read. When I peruse the WSJ on my iPad, I sometimes forget how to turn the pages, which button I should push, or where on the screen I should tap or swipe. My wife, Pammy, sometimes has to help me do that. But I still manage to get through.

No matter how difficult or aggravating the process of keeping up with current events—not to mention dealing with the news itself, which has been pretty grim the last few months!—I still make a point of doing it because I don't want to lose track of what's going on in the world.

That relates to something that has become almost a cliché about Alzheimer's patients: that they have no idea what's going on around them now, but remember details from decades ago. I'm not a neurologist but I'll suggest this: Maybe one reason Alzheimer's patients tend to slip into the past is because no one is encouraging them to stay in the present! Help your loved one stay connected; if reading is hard, they can watch TV or listen to podcasts or audiobooks.

Help us avoid becoming stereotypes

Common sense tells us that when people look better, they usually feel better. So even if it may not seem that clean clothes and personal hygiene would make a big difference to someone whose disease is advanced, I think helping your loved one look his or her best is good—for you as well as them.

I've made a concerted effort to do just that. Even though I no longer have an office to go to, I still shave every day. I know that some assisted-living facilities understand the importance of this, and they'll take the residents every week to the beauty parlor or the barber shop. I can't help but think that allowing them the dignity that comes with looking their best is a positive thing for those folks, as it is for me.

Keep us in the loop!

I may be an Alzheimer's patient, but I'm still a parent. I'm still a grandfather, a husband, a friend.

I'm fortunate to have family and friends who understand this. They don't speak about me as if I'm not there. They solicit my opinion on family matters and current events. Travis invites me to cohost most of his podcast episodes, and we really enjoy that digital time together.

While I recognize the situation is different for those in more advanced states of dementia, I still think you need to keep us included. Don't leave us out of conversations or plans, even on normal, routine stuff. Don't marginalize us. You may be surprised at how much your loved one can understand. And even if they don't seem interested or attuned to vacation plans or what's happening with the grandkids in school, I have to believe it's good for them to hear. And for you, it's a reminder that we are still present; still alive; still your father, your mother; still that person you love.

If you can hear me...

I've addressed my previous remarks primarily to caregivers. For a moment, I'd like to speak directly to those who are battling the same disease I am. Maybe you're at an early stage like me, maybe not. But perhaps your initial reaction was similar to mine.

I was angry. Very angry. As I've expressed in my journal (parts of which are excerpted in this book), I couldn't believe this was happening to me. I lashed out in frustration as my abilities became more limited; when I couldn't figure out how to put on a shirt, when I could no longer drive, when I couldn't remember how to use a TV remote or open a can.

I have since learned all that anger is a waste of time. Instead I'm trying to focus on doing everything I can to fight back against this disease, to help other people and make an impact, to take care of myself, to maintain my cognitive and physical abilities as best as I can, for as long as I can. This book project is part of that effort.

The "Why me?" stuff is understandable but leads to nothing but more misery, at least in my experience. Instead I look at my situation like this: Some of the best minds in the world are working on this disease and trying to find some kind of cure or a way to minimize its effects. Maybe I will be lucky enough to be the beneficiary of their discoveries, when they inevitably arrive. Maybe not. Either way, I'm staying as positive as I can. I don't want to be the angry, pissed-off person. I still have my moments of frustration—who doesn't? —but I'm living my life as best as I can, as productively as I can, while I can.

If you're battling this disease too, I hope you can try to do the same.

Practical advice for my Alzheimer's brethren

Here's a tip for those who are in the early stages of the disease, one that will help keep you safe and reduce a lot of the anxiety for your loved ones. I strongly recommend you always carry a cell phone or some other tracking device. For years I resisted this. But I have finally acquiesced. In my case, as I've mentioned, I still spend much of my time outdoors. I've been running the same trails for decades and can identify specific roots and rocks, but I have to admit there are times now when I pause in the middle of a run, and for a moment I don't know where the heck I am!

Whether you're out for a stroll in the neighborhood, running errands, at the mall, or wherever, it's important that your loved ones can find you if necessary. So please, swallow the old pride and take a cell phone with you when you go out. If you require assistance setting up the phone—and Alzheimer's or no, many of us older folks need help with some of this new technology—ask your grandkid!

Some pandemic perspective

As I write this, we are in the grip of the coronavirus pandemic. I'm not an infectious-disease expert, but I do know something about being restricted. Essentially, I've been confined since I was told I couldn't drive. I'm sorry that the rest of the world is now in the same boat. But I have learned to adjust, using some of the tools that I mentioned earlier, principal among them my time outdoors and my efforts to stay connected with both my family and the wider world.

You also read in this book about how Pammy needed a new kidney just before I was diagnosed. While she's doing fine, she is immunosuppressed, so we've had to be extra vigilant in our quarantine. In short, we're in this together, as we've always been. When quarantine is necessary, I can't imagine anyone I'd rather be confined with than Pammy!

In terms of the pandemic, I mentioned earlier that I was a big reader of history. Some historical context, I think, is helpful here. This is not the first time a disease has attacked the human race. Previous generations have had to beat back bubonic plague, smallpox, the so-called Spanish flu.

We can do the same.

The good news is that eventually this virus will wear itself out and the people of the world will return to their prepandemic lives. However, my Alzheimer's brothers and sisters and I will probably never be able to go back to the way things were for us, before our diagnoses. I'm not asking for sympathy here, for myself or for them; I'm just trying to provide some perspective. By the time you read these words, the epidemic will hopefully be a distant memory; a memory that I may no longer have. I hope we can use the recollections of this period wisely, to make this a better world.

In closing, to caregivers

I've written these words to you, the family member who is, to some degree, charged with responsibility for your loved one with Alzheimer's. If you're reading this, I know you're trying to do the best job possible. And because your loved one may not be able to articulate this, allow me to say on their behalf, "Thanks."

I know it's not easy. I see it with Pammy. I know that despite her cheerfulness and positive energy, it's tough to have a spouse with Alzheimer's. I can't tell her how much I appreciate what she's doing for me.

And I know if he or she could, your loved one would say the same. Thank you.

—MARK MACY,
Evergreen, Colorado

ACKNOWLEDGMENTS

ADVENTURE RACING IS A TEAM SPORT, and so is writing a book. Thanks dearly to the following people–and so many more (you know who you are)—who contributed to this project, directly or indirectly.

Dad, Mom, Amy, Wyatt, Lila, Sandy, Steve, KK, Jake, Dona, Aunt Boo, and the rest of the family—thanks for giving my life meaning. Many of you put hours and days into this dream. Patrick, you started as a colleague and became a friend; we're going to be looking back on this for years to come. Linda Konner, thanks for your hard work as our agent; your vote of confidence early on meant everything. Kevin Stevens and Donna Spurlock at Imagine/ Charlesbridge, thanks for your supreme effort and personal touch. John Hanc and John Capouya, you played a big role in getting this book off the ground, and you'll always be part of the team. Shane, Nellie, and Andrew, you were the best teammates and friends we could have asked for out there... let's split a bar sometime soon. Jari Hyatt, Erik Sanders, and Dave Mackey, thanks for the flexibility that allowed Dad and me to race together. Kevin Hodder, Lisa Hennessy, Mark Burnett, Bear Grylls, Scott Flavelle, Mindy Zemrak, Ashley Holt, and the entire *World's Toughest Race: Eco-Challenge Fiji* 2019 team—thanks for supporting us in Fiji and providing a fantastic experience. Marsh, Heather, Dr. Bob, Dean, and Dale—you are Dad's Evergreen team and extended family, and it makes all the difference.

—*Travis*

Sincere thanks to the Macy family for inviting me to help share their remarkable story. Travis, Mace, and Pam introduced me to new levels of resilience, commitment, and spirit. Your grit and positivity will inspire long after this book is done. This book is dedicated to my mom, my forever first reader. You would have loved this one.

—*Patrick*

Photograph Credits

The cover photograph and the following photographs in the sixteen-page photo insert are courtesy of Amazon Content Services LLC:

Bottom of page 1 (Team Endure)
Bottom of page 2 (Travis/Mace on bikes)
Top of page 3 (Camakau on the water)
Bottom of page 4 (Travis on bike)
Top of page 8 (Travis, Mace, Marshall Ulrich)
Bottom of page 8 (Bear Grylls and Emma Roca)
Top of page 11 (Danelle Ballengee)
Bottom right, page 12 (Stray Dogs 2019)

All other photos in the insert and the photograph of Mace and Travis on the title page are courtesy of the Macy family.